FREEDOM

· FROM ·

PAIN

The Breakthrough Method
of Pain Relief Based on the
New York Pain Treatment Program
at Lenox Hill Hospital

NORMAN J. MARCUS, M.D.
Medical Director, New York Pain Treatment Program
and Jean S. Arbeiter

· · ·

A FIRESIDE BOOK
Published by Simon & Schuster
New York   London   Toronto   Sydney   Tokyo   Singapore

FIRESIDE
Rockefeller Center
1230 Avenue of the Americas
New York, New York 10020

First Fireside Edition 1995

FIRESIDE and colophon are registered trademarks
of Simon & Schuster Inc.
Designed by Liney Li
Manufactured in the United States of America

1   3   5   7   9   10   8   6   4   2
    3   5   7   9   10   8   6   4   Pbk.

Library of Congress Cataloging-in-Publication Data

Marcus, Norman J.
Freedom from pain : the breakthrough method of pain relief,
based on the New York Pain Treatment Program at Lenox Hill Hospital /
Norman J. Marcus and Jean S. Arbeiter.
p.   cm.
Includes bibliographical references and index.
1. Intractable pain.   I. Arbeiter, Jean S.   II. Title.
RB127.M386   1994
616'.0472—dc20   93-44962
                                                            CIP

ISBN: 0-671-79892-8
0-671-51165-3 Pbk.
The ideas, procedures and suggestions
in this book are intended to supplement, not replace,
the medical advice of trained professionals.
All matters regarding your health
require medical supervision. Consult your physician before
adopting the medical suggestions in this book,
as well as about any condition that
may require diagnosis or medical attention.

The author and publishers disclaim any liability
arising directly or indirectly from the use of this book.

FOR SUZY AND FOR HANS KRAUS, M.D.,

AND

FOR SOLOMON

Contents

Author's Note

BEFORE YOU BEGIN THIS PROGRAM, IT IS IMPORTANT TO CONSULT WITH A PHYSICIAN REGARDING THE REASONS FOR YOUR PAIN. DO NOT PROCEED WITH THE STEPS OUTLINED HERE IF YOUR PAIN HAS NOT YET BEEN DIAGNOSED. REMEMBER, TOO, THAT THIS BOOK WAS NOT DESIGNED TO SUBSTITUTE FOR APPROPRIATE MEDICAL CARE; INDEED, IT IS INTENDED TO BE COMPATIBLE WITH ONGOING TREATMENT. AT ONE POINT IN THE PROGRAM YOU WILL BE ADVISED TO CUT BACK ON ANY NARCOTIC MEDICATIONS YOU MAY BE TAKING; BE SURE TO DISCUSS THE PROCESS OF CUTTING BACK WITH YOUR PHYSICIAN BEFORE TAKING ACTION.

THE PATIENTS YOU MEET IN THIS BOOK MAY SEEM FAMILIAR, SINCE UNDOUBTEDLY YOU HAVE UNDERGONE EXPERIENCES SIMILAR TO THEIRS. ALL OF THESE PATIENTS' NAMES, AND OTHER PERSONAL FACTS ABOUT THEM, HAVE BEEN CHANGED TO PROTECT THEIR PRIVACY.

"Doctor, You Have to Help Me"

The woman's voice on the telephone was low but insistent.

"If you don't help me, I'm going to kill myself."

I took a deep breath to compose myself. What I was hearing was nothing new. Months or years of living with pain *can* drive a person to contemplate suicide, so I set up an immediate appointment to see the caller, whose name was Veronica Henderson.

Veronica Henderson turned out to be a red-haired flight attendant in her mid-thirties. I could see that her face had once been attractive, but now it was drawn and painfully thin, as was the rest of her body. Her clothes hung limply, like a shroud.

When I asked Veronica to sit down, she told me that she preferred to stand because the pain was so severe.

She got to the point immediately. "I'm at the end of my rope," she said. "I want to die."

At one time, Veronica told me, she'd had a wonderful life: a glamorous job, a wide circle of friends, a chance to travel to the ends of the earth.

Then, one day, it all ended abruptly. As she was pushing a heavy cart down the aisle of a jet plane, she felt her back "pull out." Thinking the pain would pass, she went on distributing dinner trays to the passengers. By the time the plane landed, she couldn't take it anymore. She was taken to an emergency room, where doctors diagnosed a strained muscle. They prescribed muscle relaxants, heat, and bed rest. But after a few weeks in bed, Veronica felt worse. "To get around," she told me, "I had to crawl on my hands and knees."

The pain continued, long after the injury should have been healed. Veronica's sick leave lengthened into a disability leave. She went from doctor to doctor, finding relief only in the narcotic medications they prescribed. But soon she needed more and more medication, and still the pain continued.

As time went on, Veronica found it difficult to complete the simplest everyday tasks. Just washing the dishes was torture, as pain radiated through her neck, back, and arms. Gradually, she stopped trying to do things and started spending most of the day staring at television. "The pain was so bad, I couldn't do anything else anyway," she remembers. "So why bother to try?"

Without work, or any important commitments, Veronica's days became completely unstructured, a blur of discomfort, fatigue, and drugged rest.

Five years after she did "something funny" to her back while pushing the food cart, Veronica Henderson was unrecognizable to herself and to those who knew her. The morning of our interview, her weight was down to eighty-eight pounds. She walked in a forced manner, holding her arms tightly against her body. Saddest of all, as I was to learn later, her sunny personality and deep interest in the world about her had completely disappeared. Now Veronica proposed to end her existence. I knew that deep inside she didn't really want to die. What she wanted was relief.

"I can help you," I said with conviction.

For the first time, Veronica looked straight at me, and I could see a thin glimmer of hope in her eyes.

I offered Veronica Henderson an alternative to suicide and an alternative to the struggle she had been waging fruitlessly for five years. I said I would enroll her in my inpatient pain treatment program at Lenox Hill Hospital at once, ahead of the long list of names I had on the waiting list.

A Better Way to Conquer Pain
• • •

Although pain treatment programs have been in existence for several decades, what they do is not well understood.

I explained to Veronica that a pain treatment program, rather than relying on narcotic drugs and other medical treatments, relies on the ability of patients to learn to help themselves. We have learned that a variety of techniques, both physical and mental, are effective in combating chronic pain. These techniques are best learned together and then used in a coordinated fashion—an assault battery, so to speak, on the enemy. In my program we work in a very intense fashion, eight hours a day for three weeks, aiming to help people absorb skills and gain the additional self-knowledge they need to push back pain.

Veronica became one of a group of eight patients who worked, not only with me, but also with my dedicated staff of neurologists, physical therapists, psychiatrists, psychologists, physiatrists, occupational therapists, biofeedback specialists, and nurses.

Today Veronica Henderson is flying again. Her weight is at normal levels, but best of all—that easy smile has returned. "I still can hardly believe that I'm living a normal life," she told me a short time ago. "It's a miracle."

Her remark reminded me of one made by another former patient, who likened my program to a trip to Lourdes. Such statements flatter me, of course, but I know that what really happens is that people find Lourdes inside themselves. They make their own miracles.

In my program more than 75 percent of the patients improve by such measures as needing less medication, increasing their capacity to perform activities of daily living, and experiencing decreased pain. This high success rate means I've been fortunate enough to witness many turnarounds like Veronica's.

Another case worth citing is that of Toni Romano.

When I first met Toni, she was in just as much despair as Veronica. Toni was a heavyset woman who would have been attractive, but for her unkempt hair, her pallor, and the dejected expression on her face. She looked far older than her forty-something years.

For Toni, any chair, including the one in my office, was "a hotseat." She sat on the very edge, claiming that it was too painful for her to lean back. When I examined her, there was barely any place I could touch without causing her to cry out.

Toni had been the manager of a high-pressure department in a busy retail store. She took her job very seriously. "I was ready to run over there whenever they called. I had to be able to solve every problem that came up," she said.

After work Toni went home and took care of her house, which she believed she had to keep "shipshape." She was divorced and bringing up three children. She was also the mainstay of a wide circle of relatives, many of whom called her regularly for advice. In the family, she was known as the "dependable" one.

One morning Toni woke up with a nagging pain in her hip. I must have bumped into something, she thought. It'll pass. But as the weeks went by, the pain got worse.

Toni became concerned. She started visiting doctors, the number of whom would eventually reach twenty. She saw a chiropractor for six months, an acupuncturist for another six. An "arthritis specialist" gave her a shot of cortisone and put her on sleeping pills.

But things got worse, not better, as the pain spread to her other hip and other parts of her body. Toni noticed that her right thigh, from the knee to the hip, felt cold to the touch. It was difficult to raise her leg. An orthopedist gave her more cortisone.

Perhaps most disconcerting was the fact that repeated scans with magnetic resonance imaging (MRI)—undertaken to look for a herniated disk in the spine or a tumor pressing on a nerve—showed nothing. Finally the orthopedist suggested that Toni see a psychiatrist.

The psychotherapist charged $150 an hour to explore Toni's childhood. "But I was fine until this pain started," Toni finally protested. She terminated the therapy.

Her next stop was an anesthesiologist who injected the area around the nerves in her spine with an anesthetic—nerve blocks. Again, no permanent relief.

"Nothing worked, including all the drugs I was on," Toni told me.

Needless to say, Toni lost her job. She crawled into bed and stayed there, "even though I never slept." Sometimes she'd spend the entire night with her knees on the floor and her head on the bed. "My kids used to buy me things to make me more comfortable, all kinds of pillows and stuff. But nothing helped."

Toni pulled herself together for one big event—her oldest daughter's wedding. In the picture she showed me, she's standing in the midst of other relatives, wearing a blue chiffon dress and a big smile, but the strain is evident in her face.

After the wedding Toni decided to try one more doctor. Most doctors, unfortunately, don't know much about pain treatment programs—something pain specialists are fighting to correct—but this one did. He referred Toni to me.

Like Veronica Henderson, Toni had never heard of a program such as mine, but she was game.

The night she was admitted to Lenox Hill, I took her off the sleeping pills to which she had become addicted and replaced them with a minimal dose of an antidepressant. Toni slept for ten hours, the first decent night's sleep she'd had in four years.

The first week felt strange. But, bit by bit, the methods we employ made sense. By performing simple exercises, which at first she thought she couldn't do, she noticed movement returning slowly to her legs, arms, and neck. Then, after a while, the pain-fighting mental techniques, which had sounded "like make-believe" at first, caused her to feel more relaxed. She also learned how nutrition could be used to alleviate pain. And, in talking about herself and her life-style with our psychologists, she began to see how her constant quest to be perfect, to be the "dependable relative" at all times, had set her up for her condition.

Gradually she began the turning-around process. Then she progressed rapidly.

After she completed the inpatient program, Toni continued, as most of my patients do, to come in for follow-up physical therapy at least once a week for three to six months.

One morning, about two months after Toni "graduated," I walked down the hall toward the conference room where the patients and I gather for morning meetings. I saw a strange woman sitting on one of the sofas.

As I got closer, I realized that it was Toni. She had lost about fifteen pounds. Her hair was styled, there was color in her face, and she wore a fashionable pants suit. "I'm getting dressed up again," she told me. "It's fun."

I noticed that Toni was seated comfortably against the back of the sofa—only a short time ago she couldn't sit back on a chair without being in agony.

Most important, Toni was active, seeing friends, spending time with her family, shopping, going to dances. "I'm doing things I haven't done in six years," she reported. "I like people again. I'm making up for lost time."

Toni and her oldest daughter were planning to open up a dress shop. That very day they were going to sign the lease. As I watched her walk toward the elevator, without a trace of strain in her movements, I thought again of Lourdes.

"I Never Experienced Pain Like That"
• • •

Another "miracle" I think of often is the one that happened to Henry Carlson.

Henry was a construction worker at the top of his form, a vigorous two-hundred-pounder with fifteen years of experience in a most demanding kind of construction, building bridges. He had a wife, three small children, an elderly mother who lived with him, and a mortgage that was a little higher than he would have liked. Still, Henry wasn't much of a worrier because, with his skills, he was always in demand.

One day the world caved in on Henry Carlson. He was lifting a beam with two other men when they lost control of it. Henry ducked as the beam slid toward him, but it struck him in the back of the neck.

Henry remembered "feeling something real bad." Still, he could move his neck, so he figured he would simply go home and rest until the discomfort went away. Two days later Henry was totally immobilized with piercing, burning, and shooting pains all over his body. "I never experienced pain like that," he told me when I first met him.

Henry's wife drove him to the hospital, where it took him ten minutes to get out of the car. Then something happened that had never happened to Henry Carlson before. His wife saw him cry.

A scan showed a herniated disk in Henry's neck. The medical advice included bed rest, massage, and physical therapy. Henry tried them all. But, in Henry's view, nothing eased the pain, except the cervical collar that was recommended by one physician.

As the pain continued, Henry Carlson's easygoing personality began to change. Just thinking of the future was awful. He worried constantly about his diminishing savings account, and so did his wife and mother. Though they tried not to show their concern, they behaved differently toward him. Henry had always been the dominant figure in the household, making the major decisions, but now his family began to work around him. They all agreed that they shouldn't "bother" Henry: he needed his rest. The children wouldn't have dreamed of asking Henry to roughhouse with them, as he had done regularly before the accident.

Henry became increasingly isolated, not only from his family, but from the things he enjoyed. Before the accident he had been an outstanding basketball player. Now he wondered if he would ever play again, or even take long walks, or do any of the outdoor activities that were once an important part of his life.

Worst of all, Henry continued to hurt. The more he worried about hurting, the more he hurt. And the more he hurt, the more he worried about hurting. He was caught in a downward spiral, and it changed his personality.

Henry began to snap at his family and at those friends who persevered and still continued to call. On his part, Henry had stopped making phone calls to friends; he was tired of hearing the refrain, "Aren't you feeling better yet?"

Finally a stalwart friend who had seen me on the "Today" show suggested that Henry call me. He did, and after an interview and evaluation, I enrolled him in the inpatient program.

The first morning, I told Henry that I planned to wean him away from the collar, which only weakened the muscles in his neck. He would also start exercising, which he needed badly, because he had been spending most of his time lying on the sofa in the living room.

Henry glared at me. "Rest is the only thing that helps," he said emphatically. As for the collar, life would be unbearable without it.

I could see that Henry would be a tough case, and he was. At first he fought me every step of the way. The exercise made him hurt. The mental techniques made him hurt. Being without the collar for five minutes made him hurt.

But my staff and I kept trying to break through Henry's resistance, encouraging him to be just the slightest bit open.

Then the inevitable turnaround came. Henry was attending a session on body mechanics—how to perform daily activities in the most pain-free way—when a thought occurred to him: Though he couldn't do things he used to, he could still do other things.

Henry could no longer play basketball, but other sports were open to him. He could no longer roughhouse with his children, but he could play with them in other ways.

All was not lost just because he couldn't be the old Henry. He could be a new Henry who was just as good—but different.

"I've been a jerk," Henry told me as he went to work in earnest, learning to fight his pain.

After he completed the program, Henry undertook vocational retraining at a local community college. Today he works as a computer technician. His salary isn't as high as it used to be, but his wife has gone back to work, so mortgage payments can be met.

And they are thinking of moving to another part of the country where the cost of living may be lower.

Henry Carlson said good-bye to the past and openly embraced a different—though no less fulfilling—future. "There *is* life without pain," he told me. "That's what I couldn't see when I was hurting so badly."

My Promise to You
· · ·

I know that you are wondering if you will ever feel as well as Veronica Henderson, Toni Romano, and Henry Carlson do today. Let me assure you that their miracle can be yours as well, no matter what your sex, age, or background.

In my program I have patients who vary considerably in their personalities and attitudes. But the program manages to get through to just about all of them.

I have seen people who challenged me at every point, people who thought they couldn't get out of wheelchairs, people who moped and cried—I have seen those people stand up and get better!

So I am confident that wherever you are right now, you can succeed.

If you are fully committed at this point, all well and good. If you have doubts, that's all right, too. At some point, if you do what I tell you to do in this book, a breakthrough will occur.

Then you will know that your miracle has begun.

Let's begin by taking a close look at what's ailing you and why you have a condition that few people understand. It's the familiar but misunderstood term, "chronic pain."

The Truth about Chronic Pain

I've never met you, but I know you, because I've treated more than five thousand people like you who suffer from inexplicable, intractable pain.

If I saw you on the street, I might well recognize you by your labored walk or the strained expression on your face. Or I might not recognize you at all because you struggle to appear "normal" on the outside.

But inside I would be in familiar territory. Inside I would encounter an overwhelming flood of emotions that accompany chronic pain—doubt, depression, despair. If I stopped to talk with you, you might well ask me what so many others have: Why can't anyone help me?

It's amazing how long chronic pain can go on without the sufferer finding an answer to that question.

Recently, in my program at Lenox Hill Hospital, I admitted a woman who had been in pain for twenty-seven years, almost half her life. Hers was an existence of limited activity and constant pill popping. She had endured repeated operations—six in all. But still, she said, "I get no real relief."

"No real relief" is a phrase that undoubtedly applies to you, too, whether your pain has been around for months or years. Those three little words are among the saddest in the world, because they nag at you constantly. But real relief is within your grasp—at last.

What Causes Pain?

• • •

First of all, our knowledge of the physiology of pain is not complete. But we do know that pain begins when the nervous system responds to some sort of stimulus, a pinprick, a blow to the arm, or some other type of injury—a disease, for example—that causes tissue damage. The tissue damage message is conveyed by nerve fibers to the spinal cord and then to the brain. These messages are called nociceptive stimuli.

They have a purpose. They tell the brain that tissue damage has occurred. And the body reacts reflexively to protect itself. If you've put your hand on something hot, for example, you pull it away. If you've struck your finger with a hammer, you rub it. If an injury or illness seems to be severe, you seek medical attention. Pain tells us: "Go and get help." If we didn't have that signal, we could die, because we wouldn't seek to avert the damage that was taking place. Thus, acute pain, despite the suffering it creates, is an important ally.

With treatment, and in time, the tissue damage caused by an injury or an illness heals. Gradually pain diminishes. That red light telling you that something is wrong begins to fade. Finally it turns itself off completely, and you feel like yourself again.

Your pain began the same way, with an accident, an operation, an illness, or perhaps something you weren't aware of at all. You felt pain—perhaps in your lower back, abdomen, neck, or head— and you sought help. But with the passage of time the pain hasn't really diminished, though its quality may have become more "nagging" than acute. Or it may have even grown worse.

When pain continues longer than the medical profession would expect a similar condition to last, it is termed "chronic pain." Back pain, for example, is usually considered chronic when it has lasted more than three months.

The odd thing is that in most cases a medical examination will show that the body has healed. And the physiological changes that accompany acute pain—increased heart rate and respiration, among others—have returned to normal. There seems to be no substantial reason for your pain. Still, you're hurting.

If chronic pain affected only a few people, we might think they were "imagining" it in some way. But more than fifty million people in this country suffer from chronic pain. So we have to assume that chronic pain is a problem that has not yet been fully understood by the medical profession.

We have some facts. For example, Patrick D. Wall, M.D., and Ronald Melzack, Ph.D., two of the leading pain researchers in the world, have demonstrated that chronic pain is more complex than acute pain, and therefore treatment needs to address all of the contributing factors.

What we still don't know, however, is why chronic pain develops. Nor do we know why some people are affected by it and others are not. *What we do know is that chronic pain is real.* And we know what it does to people.

The Seven D's of Chronic Pain
· · ·

One of the worst aspects of the problem is that chronic pain patients are frequently treated in a way that ultimately makes them feel worse. This comes about through a series of factors I call the seven D's. Undoubtedly you've already encountered some of them:

❑ *Doctor shopping.* You travel from physician to physician, trying to find one who can "fix" your pain. You undergo numerous medical tests. You're told to rest. You're given medications. But you don't really get any better.

Perhaps a doctor finds something unusual in a scan—a herniated disk in your back, for example—and recommends surgery. But, months after the operation, the pain is still there. In fact, you may feel worse. So you undergo additional surgery. I had one patient who had been operated on seventeen times. And when he came to me, what did he want? Another operation! In our society expectations of getting "fixed" by a doctor are very strong, for both patient and doctor.

If you don't get better, your physician becomes frustrated. Without meaning to, he or she may demonstrate less sympathy, since you represent a failure of the mission to cure. You begin to feel like a pariah.

❏ **Dollars.** Not only do you feel rotten, but it's costing you big bucks to feel that way. As you seek help, the bills mount up. It's not unusual for me to see patients who have been to more than fifteen physicians and spent over $40,000. Most of these people are frustrated and pretty angry, too. And anger is an emotion that sets them up for more pain because it causes the muscles to tighten.

❏ **Drugs.** Collecting prescriptions is an almost inevitable outcome of doctor shopping, since every physician will want to offer treatment of some sort. Generally you wind up on a variety of narcotic medications. You may also be given tranquilizers. But, as your tolerance builds over time, your body tries to override the drugs' effects, and you find you need to take greater doses to get less relief. Even though you grow afraid of your increasing dependence, you keep on taking the pills, because they're the only things that give you "a little relief." You watch the clock constantly to make sure you don't miss your next medication.

❏ **Doubt.** As time goes on, doctors and relatives—more out of frustration than anything else—may suggest that perhaps nothing is "really" wrong. The implication is that your pain is all in your mind. You begin to wonder: Is it? Perhaps you can no longer trust your own judgment. You may even consult a therapist, who might tell you that you have deep-seated reasons for *wanting* all this pain. These reasons may take years—and more dollars—to analyze. In the meantime, you continue to hurt.

❑ *Disuse.* To avoid pain, you start doing less and less. You spend more time "resting," lying on your back watching television, or simply staying in bed all day. As you rest, a terrible thing happens. You lose 1 to 3 percent of body strength for *every day* that you lie in bed. Gradually your muscles become flabby. You lose calcium from the bones, too, making them more fragile. The increased weakness leads to secondary aches and pains. So you hurt more, which makes you conclude that you need more rest. You are caught in a downward spiral of pain.

❑ *Depression.* There seems to be nothing to look forward to. You feel down most of the time. You may even entertain thoughts of suicide.

❑ *Disability.* Finally, you come to think of yourself as totally disabled. You don't do very much. You're dependent on drugs. Your body is out of shape. Your self-esteem is at zero. You're totally focused on your pain. You have developed chronic pain syndrome (CPS). You are a "pain person."

What You Must Know
• • •

If you have been through the seven D's, you have developed a number of erroneous beliefs. And the most harmful of them is that you must protect your body because something is very wrong inside you. That would be a reasonable reaction to acute pain, which, as I've explained, signals an injury.

Now it is true that chronic pain, like acute pain, is a signal.

But unlike acute pain, chronic pain is *not* a meaningful signal. There is no injury. *Chronic pain is garbage in the brain.*

I know that it will take you some time to adjust to this idea. We are used to thinking in terms of the medical model that says pain means something is wrong, therefore we must do something about it. So we continue to react as if we were dealing with acute pain. We protect ourselves by stopping activity, taking medications, or crawling into bed. We hope to get better by employing these traditional responses, but we don't get better, because these measures are inappropriate for what's ailing us.

You can imagine how this idea startled Anna Gonzalez, the patient I mentioned earlier who had been in pain for twenty-seven years. For all that time, Anna had "rested" a good part of the day and depended on others to do almost everything for her. Her life was that of an invalid. And now I was telling her that she was doing exactly the wrong things, as a result of "garbage in the brain."

"It's hard to believe," she said.

But once she understood it, the garbage concept turned out to be quite comforting, because it provided the only valid explanation of why standard medical treatment had not worked.

Don't get me wrong. I'm not saying that chronic pain is nothing. Quite the contrary: I'm saying that chronic pain is *very* important—so important, in fact, that we must understand it as it really is and treat it in a way that works. Here's what we have to do:

1. We must divorce chronic pain from acute pain.

2. We have to give up the idea that there is something seriously wrong with us.

Many CPS sufferers harbor the belief that they really have cancer or some other catastrophic disease, which no doctor has managed to find as yet. So they continue to doctor shop, spend money, and fall deeper into the doldrums of the seven D's. If you've been checked out thoroughly, with appropriate examinations and medical tests, and nothing wrong has been found, you must surrender the notion that you are in great jeopardy.

Instead you must focus on understanding the truth:

1. Chronic pain poses no danger to your body.

2. Your pain *is* real. You do feel it. It's not "all in your head."

3. Chronic pain is not a moral failing. It does no good to put yourself down for having it. You should not compare yourself with other people who did not develop chronic pain after a similar illness or injury.

4. Chronic pain is not helped by "resting." Inactivity only weakens your body and sets you up for more pain.

5. Ultimately chronic pain isn't helped by painkillers, either. Instead these drugs may lower your pain threshold, and you may find, over time, that you need more of them. They also inhibit your ability to focus on overcoming pain.

6. Chronic pain does not have to be forever.

7. You don't have to know the causes of chronic pain in order to feel better.

In my program at Lenox Hill Hospital, I treat people with a variety of problems. All of them benefit from learning the same techniques for managing their pain. These techniques work with just about any type of chronic pain, including the following most commonly seen conditions:

❏ *Low back pain.* Pain in the lower back that may radiate into the buttocks and legs, making it hard to stand or sit for too long, bend over, and go up and down stairs.

❏ *Myofascial syndrome.* Pains located diffusely throughout the body, accompanied by difficulty in sitting, walking, and standing. (Pain may seem to focus on one area—the neck, for example—and then "move" to another area.)

❑ **Headache.** Pain caused either by muscular tension—so-called muscle-contraction headaches—or changes in blood vessels in the head—migraine headaches. More recent thinking, by the way, views these headaches as a continuum rather than two separate entities.

❑ **Postlaminectomy syndrome.** Pain in the back or other parts of the body following surgery for the correction of back problems.

❑ **TMJ syndrome.** Pain in the jaw, clicking of the jaw, earaches, or headaches that seem to be related to the muscles of the jaw.

❑ **Arthritis.** Aches and pains throughout the body, creakiness with movement, caused by age-related degenerative changes in the joints.

How can *one* treatment program be effective for such a variety of pains?

The reason is that chronic pain—no matter what the diagnosis or where it hurts—basically stems from the muscles.

Often a patient with low back pain will balk at this statement. "My MRI shows herniated disks," he or she explains somewhat testily. *"That's* the reason I'm in pain."

A disk is a piece of flat, fluid-filled cartilage that connects two vertebrae. The fluid acts as a "shock absorber," easing the impact of the body's weight. With time, however, the fluid may bulge at a weak point of the disk or actually be released. Then we say that the disk has become ruptured, or herniated.

Although herniated disks and bulging disks have long been blamed for back pain, there is no real evidence for this. If you took one hundred people over age forty and put them through a scan, almost half would be found to have some abnormality in the spine, including herniated disks. Most of these individuals wouldn't have any pain at all. In short, many, many more people are walking around with spinal abnormalities than with lower back pain.

Yet herniated disks continue to be targeted as the generators of back pain, and often they are treated by surgery. I think that's why

I see so many people whose back surgery was not successful. The surgery didn't get at the real factor in the pain.

The real factor is, as I said, *muscles!*

Muscles are frequently overlooked, even now. Hans Kraus, M.D., a noted figure in rehabilitative medicine and the physician who more than thirty years ago helped President Kennedy overcome back pain, said that muscles are treated as "a stepchild by the medical profession."

That still hasn't changed. Muscles are discounted because they are, well, "just muscles." Yet muscles hold the body together. They are behind every action we perform, from washing a shirt to hitting a tennis ball. No wonder muscles can be effective transmitters of pain.

The Connection of Muscles to Pain
● ● ●

There are three major types of muscle problems that cause pain:

❏ **Muscle tension** usually results from unconscious tightening up of a muscle. It occurs because we live sedentary lives and do not get rid of stress physically as our ancestors did. Most often muscle tension affects the head, back, and neck, but muscles can tighten up anyplace in the body, even in the eyelids.

Sometimes muscle tension can be quite visible. I'll look at a patient and see a jaw clenched so tightly that it can barely open. Or the brow of someone with headaches may be furrowed. Quite often though, muscle tension is not visible. And most often the individual is not aware of it.

There are many ways of releasing tense muscles, as you will learn when we get down to the techniques of the program. For now, the main thing to keep in mind is that muscle tension is the primary cause of chronic pain. This is true even if you've been told that your pain is "nerve pain." Nerves are surrounded by muscles, and when muscles tighten up they may make the nerves hurt. So, in many cases—sciatic pain in particular—muscle tension is really the cause.

❑ **Muscle spasm** occurs when a muscle contracts strongly and won't let go. When that happens you feel a sudden, intense pain, and you may be unable to move. It's like a body blow. If a person with low back pain says, "My back went out," he or she has usually experienced a muscle spasm.

❑ **Muscle weakness** may underlie both tension and spasm. It's a condition of modern life, caused by the fact that machines, rather than our muscles, do much of our work for us. Low back pain, for example, is a contemporary disease. It didn't affect our forebears at the same high rate, probably because they did a great deal of walking, running, and lifting. When your muscles are weak and out of condition, you are a target for chronic pain. Underexercised muscles may even contribute to much, if not all, of pain supposedly caused by "arthritis," as shown by the fact that many patients report feeling better with activity.

There is one more reason for chronic pain—trigger points. Trigger points are little tender nodes of degenerated muscle tissue that develop after prolonged spasm or tension and send pain throughout an area. They need to be treated by injections directly into the tender node in the muscle and also into where the muscle connects to the bone or to another muscle. An injection is followed up by three days of special physical therapy. Trigger point injections must be done by physicians who are highly experienced in this area. If your doctor thinks such injections may be appropriate for you, he or she will refer you to a specialist.

The thing to remember, though, is that muscle tension, spasm, and weakness are far more common causes of chronic pain than trigger points. And they are conditions that you personally—working at home—can do something about.

The exercises and other techniques in this program are designed to eliminate these causes of chronic pain. But before you go to work on your body, you must first go to work on your mind. You have to begin to look at your pain in a different way. That's why the first step of the New York Pain Treatment Program isn't exercise, as you might expect, but an exploration of how you experience pain, the changes it makes in your behavior, and how you must respond.

Buying into the Program

The first thing to understand is that this program is about *managing* your pain, rather than obtaining total pain relief. Pain management entails knowing how to understand and control your pain, so that it no longer controls you. It means living fully, with or without pain.

That doesn't mean the program can't make you feel better. It can indeed. Most of you will be able to diminish your pain significantly. Some of you will be able to eliminate it entirely.

But no matter what happens, you will be able to put your pain on the back burner of your life. You will be able to get back to *your* optimum level of functioning, whatever it may be.

To accomplish all this, I'll teach you several pain-fighting techniques. These techniques are effective—I can promise you that—if you give them a chance to work and if you work at giving them a chance. Sometimes people are unrealistic about pain management, expecting it to be a "quick fix." Or they want someone else, usually a doctor, to "take away" the pain.

The truth is that no one can manage your pain for you. You have to do it yourself. But I'll be with you every step of the way, and I can make your path a whole lot easier.

How the Program Works
. . .

There are two components to the New York Pain Treatment Program—the physical and the emotional. On the physical side, you'll work to increase your strength, endurance, and range of motion. On the emotional side, you'll work to jettison attitudes that encourage pain and to adopt new ones that fight pain. In fact, you'll realize that a change in attitude is your most important weapon in defeating the power of pain. You'll also learn how to cope with the stress that pain engenders and how to manage your time and activities to minimize pain.

As a result of mastering these techniques, you'll find that you can live your life as though you were pain free:

- You can love as though you were pain free.
- You can have friends as though you were pain free.
- You can have fun as though you were pain free.
- You can work as though you were pain free.

You may want relief, want it really badly, but first you must choose to function again.

By picking up this book, you've already made that choice. You said to yourself: I don't want to be a chronic pain basket case. I'm ready for something else.

I'm not telling you to forget about your pain, to ignore it, or to keep a stiff upper lip. That's not what this program is all about.

The renewed life you want comes from thinking differently about your pain and from acting differently in response to it. Learning to manage pain is a struggle that takes effort, courage, and faith —in yourself.

I know that you've been beaten down by pain, so you may not be entirely ready to trust someone who will talk tough to you. But I'm asking, as a first important step, that you open your mind to what I'm saying. This is what I ask of my patients at Lenox Hill Hospital, and they are living proof that it works.

As time goes on, and you find the program working, you'll have more and more faith in it. But to begin with, I'll settle for a small jump of faith on your part rather than a leap.

First, my ideas involve getting you to look at your pain differently, to accept a new set of premises. So I'll start by making the same request of you that I make of each new group of people when they enter our program:

Tell me what your pain is like.

I suggest that my patients say whatever comes into their minds. You might write it out on a piece of paper before you read any farther.

Now, compare your comments with those below which typically emerge in my group sessions:

- "Pain hurts."
- "Pain makes my life miserable."
- "Pain stabs at me."
- "Pain drives away my friends."
- "Pain is frustrating, difficult to live with."
- "Pain turns me into a different person."
- "Pain bugs me so that I don't think straight."
- "Pain consumes my whole life."
- "Pain is an ache."
- "Pain means that something is physically wrong."
- "Pain makes me not want to live anymore."
- "Pain changes my whole outlook on life."
- "Pain makes me irritable and angry."
- "Pain takes away my energy."

Notice that out of fourteen responses, only three—"Pain hurts," "Pain stabs at me," and "Pain is an ache"—refer to the sensation of pain. Only one, "Pain means that something is physically wrong," has to do with a medical worry. *The rest, ten out of fourteen, describe how pain affects your life and how you behave in response to pain.* I'd hazard a guess that you, too, as you tried to respond to my request, focused on the impact pain has on your emotions rather than on the way it feels.

What most distresses a person with chronic pain is what *comes* from pain—the destruction of your quality of life.

We used to think that pain was a physical entity that was often followed by an emotional reaction. Now we know that pain is a phenomena with many components that happen simultaneously. Pain and the way you perceive it—the things it "does" to you emotionally—are one and the same. Which is what can make living with pain so wearying.

Living with pain saddens you, isolates you from family and friends, makes you confused, tired, and irritable. Worst of all, it turns you into someone else—someone who can't make plans, do things for others, enjoy life on any level. "I'm not myself anymore," is a comment I hear a lot. Another is, "I can't believe the way I'm acting."

No wonder. Chronic pain is like having an invisible hammer beating up on you all the time.

The constant hammering fosters an attitude, called "catastrophizing," that strengthens and perpetuates pain. Like its nasty parent, depression, this attitude afflicts just about everyone who suffers from chronic pain.

Catastrophizing involves the continual expression of negative emotions: "I'm frustrated." "I'm depressed." "I'm defeated." It means expecting the worst, now and forever. It means turning every twinge of pain, every disappointment—physical or emotional —into a perception of disaster:

"Things are bad and getting worse."

"I'll never be able to go back to work."

"I won't have any friends left."

"This pain will destroy me."

"There's no use in trying anymore."

"I want to die."

"Why is God punishing me?"

"My body is falling apart."

"It would be better if I just got into bed and stayed there."

Catastrophizing really adds up to two words, "poor me." Or sometimes three words, "poor, poor me."

Using these words, thinking them, letting them anywhere near you, is the worst thing that can happen, worse than any sensation of pain you may feel. That's because "poor me" guarantees that the pain will continue to rule your life forever.

In large part, learning to manage pain is really a battle against that "poor me" attitude. If you can't stop catastrophizing, you can't hope to take back your life from pain.

Catastrophizing cuts off all chance of improvement because it envelops you in a persistent mass of gloom.

So you must stop catastrophizing.

I know that's more easily said than done. Like many of the actions I'll recommend in this book, this one is simple enough to say, but it takes some work to accomplish.

I know how powerful negative thoughts can be when they're linked to pain. Time after time I have seen them bring people down.

Negative thoughts are pain's allies, and they rush to defend pain's turf, pouncing each time you experience disappointment and frustration. When pain feels as if it's getting worse, catastrophizing may seem to make a lot of sense. But it's really the path of least resistance to discomfort.

So one way to cut back on catastrophizing is to *strengthen the capacity to endure discomfort.* Every activity in this program is designed, in part, to help you do just that.

Another way to diminish catastrophizing is simply to be aware that you are doing it. Sometimes catastrophic thoughts become so ingrained that they seem "natural" to us.

The next time you feel despair about your pain, try to think of the thought that triggered that feeling. Most likely you'll find that it was one of the poor me's—"I'm stuck," "I'll never be able to deal with this pain," or "My life will always be crummy."

Write down the catastrophic thought on a piece of paper. Just by writing down the words, you may be able to see how untrue they are.

Remember that a catastrophic thought is simply that—a thought, not a fact. It has no power over you unless you surrender to it. And you must fight against doing that, otherwise "poor me" will allow pain to take over more and more of your life. Each new push of the pain button in your thoughts gives pain more sway over your body, until there's nothing left in your day *but* pain. This is why I call catastrophizing "pain-button thinking."

The average person, who doesn't consider himself or herself to be in pain, experiences some element of physical discomfort every day. So a typical day might be divided up like this:

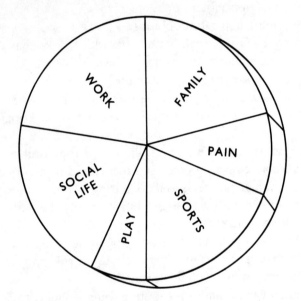

But when you suffer from chronic pain, the configuration of the pie changes. You cut back on socializing because the pain might interfere with your having a good time. You spend less time with your family because the pain keeps you from being the mother, father, or spouse you used to be. You may even leave your job because the pain keeps you from being able to work.

So now your pie winds up looking like this:

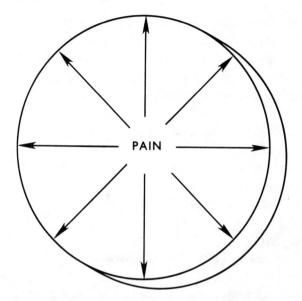

You may think that the pain "took over" because it got stronger. *But, actually, the pain got stronger because it was allowed to take over.* And step by step, as you take back portions of the pie from pain, the pain will become weaker. Getting the pie back in balance is the major task of this program—and it's something that you will be able to accomplish, gradually, with patience and courage.

Beliefs That Nurture Catastrophizing

· · ·

Catastrophizing isn't the only form of pain-button thinking. In fact, it can be just the tip of an iceberg of unfortunate beliefs that have influenced your life for too long.

Most people don't spend too much time examining their beliefs. And if you hadn't fallen victim to chronic pain, you might not have bothered to examine yours, either. But now you need to look into everything that might be making you more vulnerable to pain. So in a strange way you've been given a chance, through your pain, to learn about yourself and to change. As the wise saying goes, "God closes one door but opens another."

Look over the following list of beliefs—attitudes about life—that can actually make pain worse and check off which ones come into your mind rather frequently.

• ATTITUDES ASSESSMENT •

___I can't stand it when things don't go the way I want them to.

___There's a perfect way to solve every difficulty.

___I could never change my beliefs.

___If I don't offer help to everyone who has a problem, I'm not a good person.

___If you want to be good at what you do, your goal should be never to make a mistake.

___Self-discipline is easy for some people, but I have never been able to succeed at it.

___What I look for in all of my relationships, including work, is for people to love me.

___If I don't try to perform better than other people, I don't think I'm performing well at all.

___The bad things that happened to me when I was a child will always make my life miserable.

___I have to be in the mood to do something. Otherwise I can't do it.

___I'm not comfortable when I do something unless other people support me in it.

___You reach a point in life when you know that there's only one right way to do things.

___I can't stand it when somebody breaks a promise; he or she ought to be made to pay for it.

___Often the best thing to do in a situation is to give up.

___Before you take a chance, you should have a guarantee that things will turn out right.

___Doctors have to help me. That's their job.

___In choosing friends, I look for those who do things my way.

___I can't stand to change my feelings; I'm stuck with them.

___I organize my life to protect myself against change.

___Worrying about things that *might* happen helps me prepare for problems.

___Before I make a decision, I have to be absolutely sure that I'm making the right one.

___Someone has to have a cure for my problems.

___If there's a *possibility* that something bad will happen, it probably *will* happen.

___I can't stand it when other people don't live up to what I expect of them.

___Life should be fair.

The point of this test is *not* to score yourself. What I want you to do is discover categories that most of your beliefs fall into. So examine all of the statements you checked off, looking for the following:

❑ *"Should" beliefs.* Every time you think that events "should" happen in a certain way or that people—including yourself— "should" act in a certain way, you let yourself in for trouble. Things happen as they will; people act as they want to. Even those who love you dearly—spouses, lovers, children, relatives, and friends— will balk at being controlled in this fashion. Thus the inevitable results of "should" thinking are frustration, tension—and more pain.

❑ *Perfectionist beliefs.* We live in an imperfect world, so it's unrealistic to believe that your goal should be never to make a mistake, that there's one right way of doing anything, or that you need to know every fact before making a decision. Perfectionist beliefs like these keep you from trying anything new, such as a pain management program. If you think that you have to do everything perfectly, you're not likely to do very much at all. And you'll never find out that you can endure the discomfort of existing in an imperfect world.

❑ *"I can't stand it" beliefs.* These are among the most negative beliefs and the most untrue. The fact is that we all have a greater level of tolerance than we give ourselves credit for. When we say we *can't* stand something, we mean we would *prefer* not to put up with the discomfort it may entail. We act on our preference, not on what is actually true. Another way of saying "I can't" is to express the belief that other people have an aptitude or ability you lack, such as self-discipline. A belief like this is a real killer because it can keep you from persisting in your goal of managing pain.

❑ *Anxiety beliefs.* Chronic anxiety, like chronic pain, does not perform any useful function. If you believe that worrying is good preparation for events or that the worst is probably going to happen, you create a dysfunctional level of anxiety. It may be blocking out everything else—including the positive emotions and positive actions that can help you deal with your pain.

❑ *Dependency beliefs.* When you think that other people have to approve of you, take care of you, or provide a cure for your problems, you surrender your own wonderful ability to improve your situation. And you give in to unreality, because when it comes to chronic pain, no one can take care of you better than you can yourself. If doctors "had" to help you, you'd be cured. But the fact is, because you are reading this book, you are already past the dependent, "do it for me" part of pain control—you're about to start to take control yourself.

You may have noticed that beliefs that make pain worse have a common characteristic—their rigidity. "Should," "can't," "must," and "have to" are like steel blinders that you pull down on the world. They darken and narrow the horizon so that you can't see or feel anything but pain. But beliefs aren't the only things that can get you stuck. The way you act has a big effect, too.

Behaviors that Nurture Catastrophizing
• • •

The worst thing about chronic pain, as we've discussed, is the baggage that comes with it. Among the most cumbersome are the pieces of baggage we call "pain behaviors."

Almost everyone who has chronic pain exhibits at least some of these behaviors, which include

- walking or sitting in a hunched-over posture, as if to accommodate pain.
- walking slowly and with great effort.
- holding the body stiffly, as if to ward off an attack.
- talking in a lifeless or whiny voice.
- having a pained or vacant expression.
- groaning, moaning, or sighing frequently.
- shrugging one's shoulders to express negativity.

Pain behaviors, as you can see, are a way of saying "poor me" in body language. They are what most chronic pain sufferers mean when they say "I'm not myself anymore."

An insidious thing about pain behaviors is that you may feel as if the pain is *making* you do them. Instead you make the pain stronger by exhibiting them. Every groan and grimace assures the continued "health" of your pain.

Pain behaviors are walking depression. They poison your relationships, too, since they make other people either feel sorry for you or want to move away from you.

As with your thoughts, you must take a look at your pain behaviors if you hope to alter them.

One way to start is to ask your family and friends to describe what you look and sound like. Perhaps someone can videotape you performing daily activities. Or you can take a good look at yourself in the mirror. Watch the way you hold yourself. Walk away from the mirror, turn around, and look at yourself walking toward it.

Think about the way you move, too. If you can't straighten up "because it hurts," you're exhibiting a pain behavior. The fact is, you *can* straighten up, *even* if it hurts.

What? Is he crazy? No! You may have to strengthen your muscles—learn the exercises I will teach you—before you can fully accomplish this, but if you are motivated, you *will* straighten up.

The point is that you can act differently, no matter how you feel. A feeling is just that—a feeling. It is not necessarily reality.

Many people make the mistake of waiting for their feelings to change before they change their behavior. "I feel too crummy to exercise now. Maybe I'll feel differently tomorrow."

But if you have chronic pain syndrome, you can't afford to wait. You must change your actions now, while you work on strengthening the thoughts that bolster the new actions. You can't control the multitude of thoughts that flow through your mind, but you can consciously choose to emphasize those that are positive. And you can choose to deemphasize the pain-producing thoughts we discussed above.

Tell yourself this:

- I don't have to feel better to act as if I felt better.
- I don't have to feel better to emphasize the thoughts that can make me feel better.
- I can do what I have to do to function as well as I can, no matter how I feel.

Observe these three precepts and you'll be in for a wonderful surprise. In time your feelings will change to match your actions and your thoughts. But it doesn't work the other way around.

Inner Resources for Action
• • •

The pain treatment program at Lenox Hill Hospital is based on the principle that people can alter the way they act and think, and that there is magic in doing this. Act "as if," and "as if" will—with effort—come to be so. Human beings, just like the universe they live in, are in constant flux. You, like everyone else in the world, have the capacity to be flexible and to change.

Without being aware of it, you already have an institution—inside yourself—that can help you succeed. Donald Douglas, M.D., a prominent member of my staff, has dubbed it the First National Bank of Resources.

This bank contains the inner "capital" you need to get you through a tough situation. In fact, the resources that make up this capital have probably worked for you in the past, but you may not have been aware of them.

To fight chronic pain, however, it is necessary for you to know a lot about yourself. We ask the people in our program to consciously identify the qualities that have helped them during hard times. Just stop and think about a time in your life when you got through a situation you thought you would never get through. *You got through it!* You must have had some of these qualities:

- A positive attitude
- Determination
- Patience
- Persistence
- Endurance
- Support from family and friends
- Faith
- Courage

There are, of course, many more inner resources that you can name. Try to think about the ones that have been most effective for you. Resolve to draw on them now.

These resources are not abstractions. They are real. And they are powerful. In fact, when used in conjunction with the things you will learn in this program, they can be your most effective weapons against pain.

Remember, there are no bankers' hours at the First National

Bank of Resources. You can go there anytime, first thing in the morning or late at night.

This bank has another unusual characteristic: the more you use your resources, the more they grow. The more often you make withdrawals, the more you have in your account.

The same thing is true, by the way, of all the techniques I'll talk about. The more you use them, the more powerful they become. The more you depend on them, the more available they are to you.

As we move on to developing the program, I'd like you to keep certain principles in mind, because they will apply at each step along the way:

❏ **You will have choices.** This book will expose you to many approaches to managing your pain. Research shows that these approaches work best when they are used together. But you don't have to accept every single approach. You can be skeptical. You can even disagree with some of what I say. Buy into the techniques that are best for you, but try to keep your mind open to the others. Give them a chance to work, too. As you go on, you may discover that they are more valuable than you thought they would be.

❏ **You will believe in tomorrow.** This is not a "quick fix" program. You will notice improvements, gradually, over time. But if you stick to the program, working steadily every day, you will perceive a big difference in your ability to manage pain. It's important to be persistent and hopeful—to make constant withdrawals from the First National Bank of Resources. Step by step you will be able to take back your life from pain.

❏ **You will cope with setbacks.** Like most human endeavors, this one will not proceed steadily upward. There will be times when improvements seem to vanish, and you will think you are back to square one. Setbacks are especially difficult for people who suffer from chronic pain because they can trigger a tendency to catastrophize. When that happens, it's hard to remember that ups and downs are normal, a part of the process of getting better. So you must be prepared to fight against catastrophizing when all does not always go well.

❑ **You will encourage yourself.** You will learn how to be kind to yourself. How not to berate yourself when you mess up. How to give yourself credit for the progress you make. How to congratulate yourself for trying, day after day. How to allow yourself to feel good about small successes.

Finally, remember to accept yourself as you are and where you are right now. You can't change the past, but you can change today and tomorrow. If you work hard, you will be home free.

Pain can get better, *if you do something about it.* And that's what you are about to do.

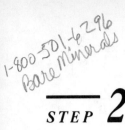
1-800-501-4296
Bare Minerals

STEP 2

Evaluating Your Pain and Your Motivation

A s you begin, you want to know how much you hurt right now and how strongly motivated you are to do something about it. Since pain is a subjective experience, this is information only you can provide.

But there are ways of "measuring" pain and of thinking about motivation. So let me show you how to get a handle on these issues.

A simple way to evaluate your pain is to use a visual analog scale (VAS), which despite its fancy name is just a plain horizontal line. Think of the line as being a kind of thermometer, with the farthest point on the left representing no pain at all and the farthest point on the right representing the most intense pain.

NO PAIN ├──────────────────────────┤ **MOST PAIN IMAGINABLE**

Now let's go to work. At the top of a piece of paper, 8½ by 11, write "Pain Evaluation Diary."

Prepare the diary to look like this:

DAY ONE.   **DATE:** _____ **TIME:** _____

1. |—————————————————————————|

On visual analog scale number one, I want you to mark the place on the line where you feel your pain is at this very minute, on day one of your fight against pain.

Take a good look at this rating, because most likely it is representative of the way you think of your pain as being most of the time.

For tomorrow, day two, prepare the diary to look like this:

DAY TWO.   **DATE:** _____

2. Waking up |—————————————————————————|

3. Midmorning |—————————————————————————|

4. Midafternoon |—————————————————————————|

5. Dinnertime |—————————————————————————|

6. Bedtime |—————————————————————————|

Complete the rest of the pain evaluation diary without looking at the first day's score. You don't have to be exactly on the minute. The idea is to get a representative sampling of your pain levels as they happen throughout the day.

If you're like most people, you probably fantasize that your pain is a monolith, a massive structure that crushes you down constantly. As you complete the scales, however, I think you'll find something unexpected. Most likely you'll see that the level of your pain, rather than being constant as you imagine, varies throughout the day.

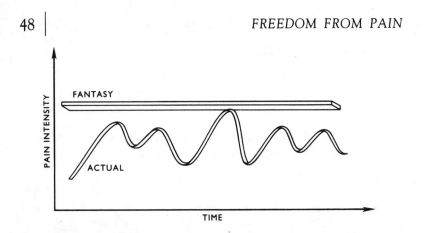

Each individual's pain doesn't have the same highs and lows, of course. But the significant thing is that there *are* highs and lows for everyone. This is a very liberating concept because it demonstrates that change is possible. You are not being crushed. You do have some breathing space, and you can take advantage of relative lows in your pain to do some of the work involved in fighting pain.

As time goes on, you will see the highs decrease and the lows increase. Bit by bit your pain will move farther to the left on the VAS.

Evaluating Your Motivation

• • •

I would like you to add one more visual analog scale to your pain evaluation diary.

|————————————————————————————|

This scale will measure something that has a big impact on your success in this program: *your motivation to get rid of your pain.*

As with measuring your pain, no one can do this evaluation but you. So write "Not Motivated" on the left-hand side of the scale and something like "Most Motivation I've Had for Anything in My Life" on the right-hand side. Then think about how motivated you are.

You'll find, I believe, that you can't "feel" your level of motivation the way you can feel your level of pain, but this check-off list should help you clarify your goals and focus on your motivation level at the same time:

• WHAT WOULD I DO IF THE PAIN WENT AWAY? •

____I'd be happy.
____I'd get a job.
____I'd feel so relieved.
____I'd be like myself again.
____I'd go back to school.
____I'd start a new relationship.
____I'd spend more time with my friends and family.

The choices here are divided into feelings and actions. If you checked off only feelings, such as "I'd be happy," "I'd feel so relieved," and "I'd be like myself again," don't rate yourself high on the motivation scale. The truth is, you're not motivated enough.

To fight pain effectively, you must have more in mind than simply to be "okay" again. You need a purpose.

Life is about wanting and doing. The phrase *I want*, followed by an action verb, has to figure prominently in your vocabulary. When I hear that phrase, I know I have a motivated patient. Here are some of the action "wants" I've heard recently:

- I *want* to go back to work.
- I *want* to start socializing again.
- I *want* to play tennis.
- I *want* to have sex again.
- I *want* to see that hit show on Broadway.
- I *want* to go out dancing.
- I *want* to learn carpentry.

You get the idea. This is the time to think about what you really, truly want out of life. Visualize yourself doing the things you want to do. Commit yourself to being able to do them.

If you can't even imagine what you would want to do, begin to work on developing some vocational and personal goals. You can't wait until you feel better to have the goals. It works the other way around—you need the goals to feel better.

But let's start with where you are at this moment. Mark your current motivational level on the visual analog scale. Then put your pain evaluation diary in a place where you can find it easily.

We'll be doing more work in the diary later on, at a time when you should be noticing changes in your levels of pain and motivation. These changes will occur as you do the work of the program, starting with the new things you'll learn about the way you relate to your body.

Interacting with Your Body

I'd like you to do something for me right now. Put down this book, walk into the kitchen, and pour yourself a glass of water.

Now think about that experience.

Were you aware of getting up out of your chair?

Walking across the room?

Pouring the glass of water?

Settling back onto your chair?

If you're like most people, you probably didn't think about your *movements* at all. You stood up, poured the water, and picked up this book again without noticing how you used your skeletal muscles to get up and down and go back and forth. Rather than concentrating on your body, you may have thought, Why is he asking me to do this silly thing?

In our civilization we tend to be aware of what we're *thinking,* not how we're moving.

To us a movement is just a way of getting something done. Whether we accomplish a task in a smooth, easy fashion or a jerky, rough one, it's all the same to us. And lots of us get into the habit of putting unnecessary strain on our bodies, without being aware that we are doing anything harmful.

Many people can operate this way all their lives and get away with it. But when you're in chronic pain, you can't, because rough use of your body tenses the muscles and increases pain. *You must become aware of how your body works so that you can use it in the most pain-free manner.*

The activities in this chapter are designed to help you become familiar with the effects of moving various groups of muscles.

To learn to move in the right way, we must *feel* what we're doing and let the feeling become committed to kinetic memory—the part of our memory banks that records the way we move. *Without awareness, we cannot distinguish between a good movement and a harmful one.* But, usually, we don't concentrate on our bodies long enough to become aware. As a consequence we miss sensing the subtle, inner signals that can help us.

Moshe Feldenkrais, the movement expert on whose work much of the material in this chapter is based, wrote that a person without body awareness is like a carriage being driven by a sleeping coachman. The carriage goes off in all directions because the horses—the muscles—are not being managed properly.

Right now your body is like that carriage. To get the carriage moving better, you need to reorganize and strengthen your muscles. It's time for you, the sleeping coachman, to wake up. But first you have to learn a technique that will make it easier for you to *feel* what your muscles are doing.

Where Body Awareness Begins
· · ·

You may be surprised to learn that an important part of body awareness is the way you breathe.

Many people with CPS are scared to death to breathe. They are so frightened of feeling pain that they take small, tight breaths. Shallow breathing, though, serves only to increase tension because it tightens the muscles. And tight muscles mean more pain.

Breathing deeply and consistently can break this pattern. The deepest breathing—diaphragmatic breathing—relaxes the muscles.

By consciously encouraging diaphragmatic breathing, you become tuned in to the way your muscles react to changes in breathing. *So to explore your body, you must first learn this valuable technique.*

Many people think that deep breathing is easy enough, simply a matter of taking a deep breath. So try doing that now.

Did your chest move in and out? Did your rib cage and shoulders move upward? If these things happened—and they probably did—you are breathing predominantly with your *chest*, not your *diaphragm*. This is the way we normally breathe in our culture. We are used to it, but it is not the most efficient, relaxing—or pain-fighting—way to breathe.

You want to breathe so that your belly expands, while your chest remains still. To practice doing this, put your hands on top of your belly or lift them over your head. Relax your shoulders, breathe deeply without moving your chest, and observe that your belly pushes out. Now practice the same thing without putting your hands on your belly or over your head. Remember to keep your chest and shoulders still. The only thing that should be moving is your belly, slowly and gently. This movement is actually the diaphragm sucking air in and pressing air out of your lungs in the most effective manner.

To really learn diaphragmatic breathing, you don't have to think about it all the time. Just practice taking a few breaths in this manner every hour or so. After a time you will find that this breathing is becoming more natural to you. At some point it may become as natural as it is for little babies. And as you do more and more of it, you'll find that you feel less hurried and less tense. Your concentration will improve. And you should begin to experience less pain.

Preparing to Explore Awareness
* * *

When you understand how things work, you do them better. So think of body awareness as a lesson in understanding. You will learn how to understand and, consequently, how to redirect the way you use your muscles *by moving*. This involves a special kind of moving that requires you to concentrate hard on what you are doing.

So, for starters, you need a quiet place in which to work. No radio or television. No friends or family members chatting nearby. You want to be able to listen—really listen—to your body.

Once you have selected a suitable space, draw the blinds or curtains so that the room is semidark. Make sure the temperature is comfortable. Avoid places where air-conditioning or heat will be blowing straight on you.

You will need an exercise mat to work on. Also have a pillow on hand. A pillow is required for some of the movements but you can use one all the time if you'd be more comfortable. Wear comfortable, loose-fitting workout clothing, the kind you usually knock about in. Work in your stocking feet.

Eda Yuhjtman, the creative physical therapist who has adapted the body awareness movements for our program, asks patients to keep these general ideas in mind before they begin to work:

❑ **You need to pay attention.** You will read the words *notice* and *feel* in the instructions for these movements, and you must concentrate on what you are doing. Otherwise the movement will not be transmitted to your kinetic memory. It's a good idea to have someone read the instructions to you the first few times you do the movements. If you prefer, you can record the instructions and play them back as you work.

❑ **You need to organize mentally.** Before you perform a move-ment, read all the instructions. Think about them. See yourself moving. Then start to move.

❑ **You need to counter the "pull-back response."** If you feel an increase in symptoms while doing a movement, you may inter-pret it as a signal to stop. Try not to give in to this urge to quit. These movements cannot hurt you physically. On the contrary, they will help to make you better.

❏ **You need to "let go"**—loosen your muscles—when instructed to do so. You can help yourself let go by imagining that you are lying in a particularly comfortable spot, on soft, warm sand, for example, or on a pile of down pillows. Later on in this program, you'll see how this sort of visualization can assist with several types of relaxation techniques.

Prepare for body awareness by telling yourself the following:

1. I am not going to be afraid.

2. I am going to concentrate.

3. I am going to work carefully.

4. I am going to think *and* feel.

5. I am going to be patient.

With these attitudes in place, you are ready to explore your muscular self.

Begin by getting down on the floor—very slowly and carefully. If necessary, hold on to a chair or another piece of stable furniture for support. Next, slide onto the mat—slowly—until you are lying down. Be certain that you are comfortable before you start to work.

EXPLORATION #1:
Feeling the way your body is organized.

___

1. Lie on your back with arms outstretched slightly and legs straight and slightly apart.
___*Notice* how your shoulders feel. Find the place where they are most comfortable. For most people, it's when the arms are halfway between the waist and shoulders with palms turned up.
___*Think* about what it feels like to be comfortable.

2. Breathe deeply and let your body feel heavy on the floor. Mentally scan your body from head to toe. Think of how it is organized.

___*Feel* which portions of your head, shoulders, upper back, lower back, and legs are touching the floor.

___*Notice* which portions are not touching the floor.

___*Remember* the contact points and the spaces.

EXPLORATION #2:
Feeling how a change in position affects other parts of your body.

1. As before, lie on your back with arms outstretched slightly and legs straight and slightly apart.

___*Notice* how much of your lower back is touching the floor.

2. Keeping your feet on the floor, bend your knees, one at a time, inhaling deeply and then exhaling.

___*Feel* that more of your lower back now touches the floor.

___*Notice* how much space there is between your neck and the floor.

3. Slowly lift your arms up toward the ceiling (while inhaling) and bring them down to the floor, reaching toward the wall behind your head (while exhaling).

___*Feel* that there is less space between your neck and the floor when your arms are moving overhead.

___*Feel* your rib cage move up and your chest expand.

4. Bring your hands back down to your sides.

___*Feel* that there is more space between your neck and the floor.

5. Repeat the movement four times.

___*Move* slowly and smoothly. Smoothness of movement is more important than size.

___*Match* your breathing to the timing of the movement.

6. Straighten out your legs, one at a time.

___*Feel* that more of your lower back touches the floor.

___*Notice* that the closer your lower back and neck get to the floor, the less tension you feel. That's because the muscles have lengthened and become less tight. So position can release tightness.

_____*Think* about how it *feels* when tightness is released.

Before you do the next movement, roll your head gently from side to side three times, exhaling as you roll to the side and inhaling when you come back to center. This serves to release tension around your neck.

EXPLORATION #3:
Feeling shifts in the connection between pelvis and head.

1. Lie on your back with arms outstretched slightly, knees bent, and feet on the floor, shoulder width apart.

2. Remaining on your back, slowly drop both knees to the right (while exhaling).
_____*Notice* that the right buttock becomes heavier while the left buttock rises off the floor.

3. Return knees to the center (while inhaling).

4. Lower knees to the left (while exhaling).
_____*Notice* that the left buttock becomes heavier while the right buttock lifts off the floor.

5. Return knees to the center (while inhaling).

6. Gently rock your knees to the right and left four times, exhaling and inhaling.
_____*Move* slowly and smoothly.
_____*Match* your breathing to the timing of the movement.
_____*Let go* between movements.
_____*Control the pull-back response.* If you feel any discomfort, decrease the size of the movement. Find a range within which you feel comfortable, even if you can move only a little bit. *But keep moving.*

___*Notice* the rotation of your pelvis. Your knees may be leading the movement, but the pelvis is its center.

___*Mentally* follow the path of the movement: knees, pelvis, rib cage, shoulders, neck, and head.

___*Think* about how much you have to move to get the optimum effect. Try not to move any more than that. Remember how it *feels* not to overdo.

EXPLORATION #4:
Feeling ribs open and close.

1. Lie on your right side with your right arm outstretched on the floor, on a line with your body. Rest the right side of your head on your right arm and your left arm on your left hip.

2. Lift your left arm over your head and touch the floor (while inhaling), as if you were drawing a rainbow.

___*Notice* that the ribs on your left side open.

3. Return your left arm to the starting position (while exhaling).

___*Notice* that the ribs on your left side close.

4. Repeat the movement four times.

___*Move* slowly and smoothly.

___*Match* your breathing to the timing of the movement.

___*Control the pull-back response.*

___*Feel* the balance between the opening and closing of your ribs.

___*Think* about how the parts of your body are organized to work together.

5. Carefully roll over on your left side and perform the movement four times, making the rainbow with your right arm.

Before you do the next movement, lie on your back with your feet slightly apart. Gently rotate your head from side to side three times, exhaling as you roll to the side and inhaling as you return to the center.

EXPLORATION #5:
Feeling stomach muscles shorten and back muscles lengthen.

_____

I. Lie on your back with arms outstretched slightly, knees bent, feet on the floor and slightly apart.

2. Put your left hand under your head, bring your right knee toward your chest, and hold it with your right hand, keeping all five fingers together.

3. Bring head and right knee toward each other (while exhaling), focusing your eyes on your knee. Do *not* force your head up with your hand. Do *not* attempt to do a situp.
___*Feel* that your abdominal muscles shorten.
___*Notice* that your lower back presses down on the floor as muscles expand.

4. Lower head to floor and return right hand and knee to starting position (while inhaling).
___*Notice* that your abdominal muscles expand.
___*Feel* that pressure is relieved in your lower back.

5. Repeat the movement four times.
___*Move* slowly and smoothly.
___*Match* your breathing to the timing of the movement.
___*Let go* between movements.
___*Control the pull-back response.*
___*Focus* on the contraction and expansion of muscles.

6. Keep knees bent, feet on the floor. Put your right hand under your head, bring your left knee toward your chest, and hold it with your left hand, keeping all five fingers together.

7. Repeat the movement four times, this time bringing head and left knee toward each other.

EXPLORATION #6:
Feeling how body organization improves quality of movement.

With your head and neck supported by a pillow, lie on your right side. Your legs should be slightly bent, with the left leg a bit out in front of your right. Be sure that your head and neck are supported by the pillow. Stretch your arms straight ahead, shoulder level, with hands resting palm on palm, left palm on top.

I. Move left arm up toward the ceiling and down to the floor behind you (while inhaling). Follow your hand with your eyes so that your head and neck rotate as you move your arm.
____*Notice* that your head, eyes, neck, shoulders, ribs, and spine organize together in a common rhythm.

2. Return left arm to the starting position (while exhaling).

3. Repeat the movement with your left arm three times, inhaling and exhaling and rotating your head, neck, and trunk as well as your arm. Direct the movement with your eyes.
____*Move* slowly and smoothly.
____*Match* your breathing to the movements.
____*Control the pull-back response.*
____*Notice* that integrating the components—head, neck, arm, and trunk—produces a smoother movement.
____*Let go* after completing the series.

4. Roll over onto your left side. Do the movement four times using your right arm.

Before you do the next movement, lie on your back with your legs straight and slightly apart. Gently roll your head from side to side a few times, exhaling as you roll to the side and inhaling when you return to center.

EXPLORATION #7:
Feeling muscles get stronger.

Lie on your stomach with your face down and your arms extended on the floor past your head.

1. Stretch your right arm out, reaching away from your body, and stretch your left leg, toe pointed (while inhaling).
——*Feel* back muscles contract.

2. Relax right arm and left leg (while exhaling).
——*Feel* back muscles expand.

3. Repeat the movement, this time stretching your left arm and right leg.

4. Lift right arm and left leg a bit off the floor (while inhaling), keeping your head on the floor.

5. Return right arm and left leg to floor (while exhaling).

6. Repeat the movement two times.
——*Move* smoothly and easily.
——*Match* your breathing to the movement.
——*Let go* after each movement.
——*Control the pull-back response.*
——*Notice* the strengthening of your back muscles as they contract and expand.

7. Repeat the movement two more times, this time lifting and then lowering left arm and right leg.

Before you do the next movement, lie on your back with knees bent and hands holding your knees. Bring knees up to your chest and rock from side to side four times, breathing evenly as you do so. Feel how the floor massages your back. Slowly straighten your legs back down to the floor, one at a time.

EXPLORATION #8:

Observing that movement facilitates movement.

1. Lie on your back with arms outstretched slightly, knees bent, and feet on the floor and slightly apart.

2. Slowly drop both knees to the right (while exhaling).

3. Return knees to the center (while inhaling).

4. Slowly drop both knees to the left (while exhaling).

5. Return knees to the center (while inhaling).

6. Gently rock knees side to side four times, exhaling and inhaling.
____*Move* slowly and smoothly.
____*Match* your breathing to the timing of the movement.

7. Let go.
____*Notice* that it's easier to do this movement now than it was earlier (Exploration #3).
____*Remember* that the more you move, the easier it becomes to move.

EXPLORATION #9:

Rechecking your body.

1. Lie on your back with arms outstretched slightly and legs straight and slightly apart.

2. Breathe deeply, slowly, and easily.
____*Feel* that your rib cage moves up and down with greater ease.
____*Notice* that deep breathing feels more "natural" now than it did when you began this session.

3. Think back to Exploration #1. Try to remember which portions of your head, shoulders, upper back, lower back, and legs were touching the floor then.

——*Feel* that more of your body is probably contacting the floor now. That means you have already succeeded in relaxing your muscles and lengthening them.

——*Notice* that your shoulders seem to be wider.

——*Remember* how it feels for your muscles to be more relaxed and expanded.

You have concluded your first body awareness session. Follow these instructions in getting up from the floor: Lying on your back, bend your knees, one at a time. Carefully roll toward your stomach and get up in one of the following two ways.

Method One. Get up on your hands and knees. Stay there for a moment, looking straight ahead, to prevent dizziness. Then get on one foot, drop your head, lift up your pelvis, and get on the other foot, still keeping your hands on the floor and both knees slightly bent. From this bent-over position, slowly uncurl your back, one vertebra at a time—from bottom to top—and get up.

Method Two. (This method is better for those who had more difficulty moving.) Get up on your hands and knees. Stay there for a moment, looking straight ahead, to prevent dizziness. Then bring one foot forward so that you are balanced on one knee and one bent leg. Straighten up your trunk to a vertical position. Place your hands on the knee of your bent leg and, pushing from your legs, rise to a standing position. If necessary, support yourself on a stable chair or piece of furniture.

Observing Your Posture
• • •

Stand with your feet apart and pay attention to establishing the correct posture. Eda Yuhjtman asks our patients to think back to the way they felt when they were lying on the floor with shoulders wider, muscles lengthened, and had a good idea of where the parts of their bodies were located. That's the way you should be standing now—wider, taller, and well put together. Your knees should be a bit bent, not "locked." (Knees are shock absorbers. If they're straight, they can't do their job.) Make sure your weight is distributed equally between the heels and the balls of your feet. All of your toes should be touching the floor, so that you maintain balance.

You should feel "lighter" than you did before you started this chapter and better aligned. Even if you notice that you're only a bit lighter, appreciate what you've accomplished. Congratulate yourself. Small changes are the stuff of which success is made.

If you don't feel any changes now, don't be discouraged. You may later on during the day, and you certainly will in time. *The important thing is that your body has begun to redirect itself.*

Your job is to continue the process by performing these movements twice a week for at least two months. (Some patients in my program come back for weekly sessions for a year.) But don't begin body awareness until you're ready to commit yourself to following through. Better not to do it than to do it halfway. Remember that *whether* to commit and *when* to commit are choices you have. This is true for all of the techniques in this program.

If you decide to go ahead, you'll find that your kinetic sensitivity expands rather rapidly. Right now you are like an iron ball. If a fly landed on you, you wouldn't notice anything at all. But if you were a feather, you'd notice a difference immediately. Body awareness means being able to feel things as a feather would.

Obviously you can't turn yourself into a feather, but you can become more attuned to your body's need to move properly. You'll find, as you continue to work on body awareness, that the movements are extremely subtle, and you will notice something new and valuable about them every day. *Noticing* is the key to becoming more like a feather and less like an iron ball.

Remembering Principles of Movement
· · ·

In addition to noticing, you need to translate what you have learned into your daily life. I'll expand on this in a later chapter on the physics of movement, when you'll also have other techniques under your belt that you need to perform everyday tasks. For now, however, here are some general things to keep in mind about moving:

· DO ·

- breathe so that your belly expands while your chest remains still.
- scan your body and realign your posture when necessary.
- move smoothly and easily.
- keep your body in balance.
- use the largest muscles—the buttocks, thighs, and abdominals—to do most of the work.
- avoid superfluous efforts.

· DON'T ·

- strain or force a movement.
- constantly raise your shoulders.
- walk without swinging your arms.
- walk with a limp.
- lock your knees.
- sit or walk in a hunched-over position.

In sum, *remember to keep in mind what you are doing.* Always concentrate on how you are moving and the best way to move. Put your thoughts into your body and your body into your thoughts.

Responding to the Pull-Back Response
· · ·

A few words about controlling the pull-back response—the urge to quit—which tends to become reflexive when you suffer from chronic pain. You can overcome it by being aware of the catastrophic thoughts provoking the response:

- Oh, my God! I felt a shooting pain. I know I've done something terrible to my body.
- This is too hard. I'll never be able to succeed at this. I'll just have to be in pain forever.
- If I keep this up, something awful will happen. I'd better stop now.

You also have to pay attention to those nasty "poor me" thoughts:

- Why should I have to do these movements? Nobody else I know does. Poor me.
- I shouldn't be expected to do something that makes me feel uncomfortable. Poor me.
- How did I get myself into a pickle where I have to listen to this guy? Poor me.

These thoughts lose their power when you remember that *they are just thoughts*. You can think them if you choose, but you can think more positive thoughts, too. You can go about your business of moving and getting better even when you are feeling apprehensive.

As you act, the tyranny of "pain-button thinking" will diminish. As you continue to act, the movements will become more comfortable. The more comfortable movement becomes, the more motivated you will be to do more of it. The process begins with action and ends with greater action, just like a spark igniting an engine.

And the important thing is that by acting, you not only strengthen yourself physically, you strengthen yourself mentally as well.

All of this happens gradually—in time.

And in time you add more and more pain-fighting techniques to your arsenal, including the important set of simple exercises presented in the next chapter.

Relaxing and Strengthening Your Body

Earlier I told you that your pain probably stems from the three most common muscle problems: tension, spasm, and weakness. Whether you suffer from one or all of these conditions, I'm going to teach you a basic way to correct the situation: the right type of exercise.

By "the right type," I mean exercises that relax and then limber your muscles—move them within a comfortable range—so that tension is released and strengthening ultimately takes place.

All of this happens slowly and gently, words that run counter to the popular notion of exercise as hard work. If you have that notion, you must give it up. As a CPS sufferer, you need to exercise in a way that's suited to people in pain. *You do not need*

- a workout in which you jump up and down and drive yourself to the limit. "No pain, no gain" may sound pretty good when you're not in pain all the time. But when you are, you don't need to hurt even more.
- a workout in which you make powerful movements. "Moving tough" at this point can only increase your pain.
- a workout in which you concentrate on only one part of your body, such as your stomach.
- a workout that makes you feel guilty all the time because you

can't meet its expectations. People with CPS walk around with enough guilt.

The fact is, you don't need a work*out* at all. What you need is a work-*in*. A work-*in* combines your *inner* knowledge of how your body moves—already gained from your attention to body awareness —with simple exercises that gradually increase the strength *inside* your muscles. Many people are surprised by how simple these exercises actually are and how quickly they are committed to memory. But the simplicity is deceptive because *these exercises are powerful.* They do just the amount of work that is needed to fix the problem.

The following ten exercises were developed specifically for people with chronic pain. They are based on the work of Hans Kraus, M.D., the noted expert on back pain and the first to recognize the importance of muscles in treating CPS.

This routine is so effective that Michael Fox, one of my physical therapists, dubbed it the "holy half hour." That's the amount of time—give or take a few minutes—that it takes most people, *working properly.*

As with most things "holy," these exercises have certain requirements:

1. *Devotion.* If you choose to commit to this routine, you must perform it *at least* once every day. There is no one best time, but many people find that first thing in the morning is most effective. Exercise can relieve early morning achiness and set the course for a more pain-free day.

2. *Belief.* You must believe that movement is good for you and will ultimately make you better. You also have to believe in another important component of the exercise program—diaphragmatic breathing—breathing so that your belly expands while your chest remains still—with which you are familiar from your body awareness routine. You must

- take deep breaths when instructed to do so.
- let go—exhale or loosen your muscles—when instructed to do so.

Deep breathing greatly increases the power of the exercises. And it also aids in letting go of tension.

3. A *dedicated space.* As with the body awareness movements, you need a quiet, comfortable place in which to work. It's best to work in the same place every day, so that you're encouraged to keep up the routine.

In addition to appropriate space, you also need

- loose-fitting exercise clothing.
- an exercise mat.
- a pillow, if you think your head needs support.
- a straight chair, with no arms, for one of the exercises.

It's best to work without shoes (even though the following illustrations show people in light gym shoes) and to keep the temperature in the room at a level that is comfortable for you.

Remember, too, that if you feel any discomfort, you should modify the movement, but stop only if you cannot avoid creating pain.

As you exercise, you again need to counter the pull-back response. In the preceding chapter I explained how catastrophic thoughts set off that response. But "pain behaviors" can trigger it, too. So before you start to work, let's put a "not allowed" sign on the following behaviors:

- Sighing
- Groaning
- Scrunching up your face
- Gritting your teeth
- Expletives

I know that it can be difficult to stop doing these things. Patients frequently tell me, "I can't help it." They believe that expressing the pain somehow releases it and makes them feel better. *But acting as if you are in pain makes you feel worse.* It reinforces your belief that you are a sick and suffering person. It makes the world look at you that way, too, which ultimately adds to your depression. The result is an undermining of your determination to manage your pain and increase your ability to function.

That's why you must concentrate on being aware of how you act. If you act *as if* you feel no discomfort, the discomfort will lessen. Your actions can put you in control. This isn't easy to do, but you *can* do it, and with greater ease as time goes on. Think about this:

- You have a choice about how you want to act.
- You have a choice about how successful you are going to be.

With these concepts in mind, you are ready to begin the exercise routine or, I should say, the exercise circle, because this routine begins with relaxation, limbering, and simple stretches, builds up to slightly more complicated stretches, and ends by working back to the starting point.

Let me say that these ten exercises are also deceptively simple. Though it's easy to regard them as "baby stuff," they are just the opposite; they are exactly what a grown-up like you needs because they were created specifically for pain problems. So take them seriously. If possible, have someone read the instructions to you the first few times you do them. Otherwise, read all of the instructions through carefully before you begin. You need to concentrate hard while you do the exercises, even though they seem to be easy.

A word of caution: If you can do all of the exercises without feeling significant discomfort, fine. But if you are not used to exercising, and you find the last three exercises uncomfortable, do only the first seven for four weeks. Then add the next three, one at a time. Don't add an additional exercise until you can do the previous one without pain.

Keep in mind, too, that much of the effectiveness of the routine depends on its circularity, so be sure to do the exercises in the order in which they appear, and always finish by working your way back to the beginning.

• THE HOLY HALF HOUR •

Get down onto the exercise mat slowly. If necessary, hold on to a piece of furniture for support.

Then lie on your back, with arms at your sides, feet on the floor, and knees bent. Take a deep breath and let it go. Repeat two times.

Mentally prepare to do all exercises slowly and gently. As with the body awareness movements, concentrate on achieving a smooth motion. Do not bounce. Move only as much as it is possible for you to move comfortably.

EXERCISE #1:
Muscle Relaxers

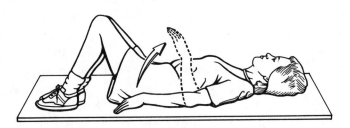

Lie on your back with your arms at your sides, feet on the floor, knees bent and slightly apart.

1. Take a deep breath and let it go.

2. Stretch your fingers and let them go. Repeat one time.

3. Tighten your fist and let it go. Repeat one time.

4. Take a deep breath and let it go.

5. Tighten your fists, forearms, biceps, chest, stomach, calves, and thighs. Take a deep breath and let everything go. Repeat one time.

6. Bend one arm at the elbow and let it drop gently back to the floor. Then bend the other arm at the elbow and let it drop gently back to the floor.

EXERCISE #2:
Shoulder Shrug

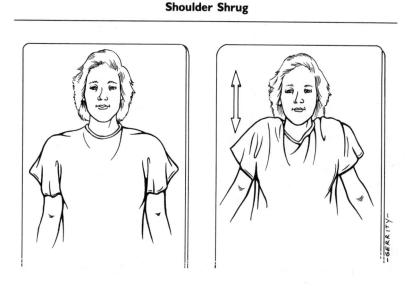

Lie on your back with your arms at your sides, feet on the floor, knees bent and slightly apart.

1. Shrug your shoulders as far up as you can and let them go. Repeat two times.

2. Take a deep breath and let it go.

EXERCISE #3:
Head Roll

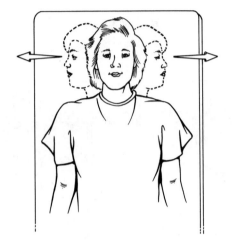

Lie on your back with your arms at your sides, feet on the floor, knees bent and slightly apart.

1. Roll your head gently to one side and back to center. Then roll it to the other side and back to center.

2. Roll your head gently back and forth about six times.

3. Take a deep breath and let it go.

EXERCISE #4:
Single Knee Flex

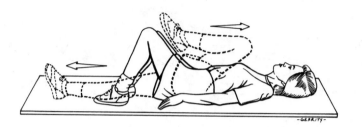

Lie on your back with your arms at your sides, feet on the floor, knees bent and slightly apart.

1. Take a deep breath and let it go.

2. Bring your right knee toward your right shoulder and return to the starting position.

3. *Slide* your right leg down to the floor and then *slide* it back to the starting position.

4. Bring your left knee toward your left shoulder and return to the starting position.

5. *Slide* your left leg down to the floor and then *slide* it back to the starting position. Repeat the entire exercise two times, alternating legs.

6. Take a deep breath and let it go.

EXERCISE #5:
Leg Extension

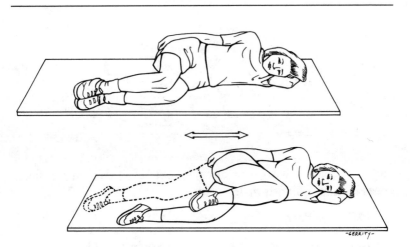

Lie on your right side in the fetal position, knees bent at a ninety-degree angle, with your right hand under your head and your left arm resting lightly on your left hip.

1. *Slide* your left knee toward your shoulder.

2. *Slide* your left leg slowly down your right leg toward the floor until it's straight. (Feel the heaviness of your left leg as it moves.)

3. *Slide* your left leg back to the starting position. Repeat the entire exercise two times.

4. Take a deep breath and let it go.

5. Carefully roll over onto your left side, assume the fetal position, and repeat the exercise three times, using your right leg.

6. Take a deep breath and let it go.

EXERCISE #6:
Buttock Tightening

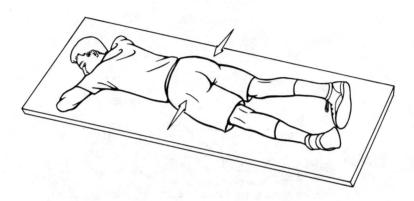

Lie flat on your stomach with your cheek resting on folded hands and your toes pointing inward.

1. Take a deep breath and let it go.

2. Tighten your buttocks and let them go. Repeat two times.

3. Take a deep breath and let it go.

EXERCISE #7:
Double Knee Flex

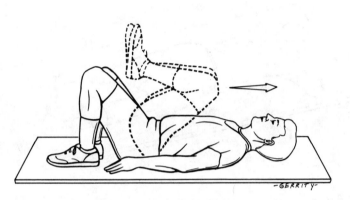

Lie on your back with your arms at your sides, feet on the floor, knees bent and slightly apart.

1. Take a deep breath and let it go.

2. Bring both knees toward your shoulders. Return to the starting position. Repeat two times.

3. Take a deep breath and let it go.

EXERCISE #8:
Cat Back

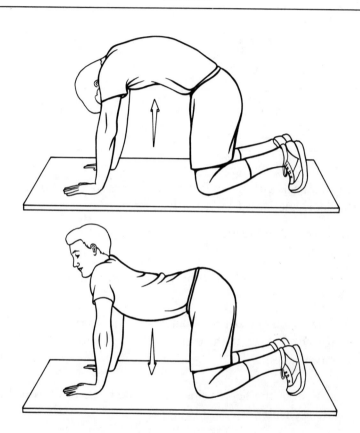

Get on your knees with your upper body balanced on your hands.

1. Lower your head, then slowly round your back, like a cat, vertebra by vertebra, bringing your buttocks in.

2. Slowly lift your head and push out your buttocks, uncurling your back, to create a "U shape." Repeat entire exercise two times.

EXERCISE #9:
Half Situps

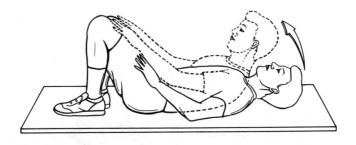

Lie on your back with hands resting on the base of your thighs, feet on the floor, knees bent and slightly apart.

1. Take a deep breath.

2. Exhale, lifting your head and shoulders slightly off the floor and slowly moving your fingers up your thighs. *Do not attempt to do a full situp.*

3. Lower your head and shoulders to the floor while moving your fingers back down to the base of your thighs. Repeat the entire exercise two times.

Get up from the floor, using one of the methods described in the previous chapter.

EXERCISE #10:
Forward Bending from a Chair

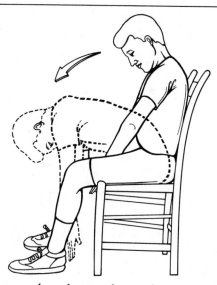

Sit on a straight, armless chair with your legs apart and arms resting easily on your inner thighs. Let your chin rest on your chest and your shoulders sag.

1. Bending forward loosely from your waist, drop your hands and head toward the floor as far as you can go.

2. Come back up to the starting position, straightening your back as you do so. Repeat the entire exercise two times.

Repeat Exercise #9.
Repeat Exercise #8.
Repeat Exercise #7.
Repeat Exercise #6.
Repeat Exercise #5.
Repeat Exercise #4.
Repeat Exercise #3.

Repeat Exercise #2.
Repeat Exercise #1.

To complete the routine, stay on your back and breathe deeply, in and out, for a few moments. You should be feeling relaxed and, as with the body awareness movements, you should also be feeling lighter and wider. In time you will also feel stronger.

Remember to get up from the floor slowly and carefully, following one of the two methods described in the previous chapter. Be sure to use a stable piece of furniture for support, if need be.

If You Feel Achy
· · ·

Some people report feeling achy after they complete the first few sessions of exercise.

If that happens to you, remember that there is no danger of injury. The achiness stems from using muscles that may not have been used for a long time. What you're experiencing is the "good pain" of getting things moving again.

If you think about it, you can probably recognize the difference between "good" and "bad" pain. The "good" achiness makes you feel as though you've accomplished something. Most likely it will soon go away, to be replaced by increased feelings of physical and mental well-being. If the achiness comes back from time to time, that's all right, too. Setbacks, in the form of various aches and pains, are normal.

One way to cope with achiness is to attribute what you feel to change rather than to pain. You can think, Something new is happening to my body, rather than, Something's wrong! I'm hurting.

Other coping methods include a refusal to catastrophize or to engage in pain behaviors.

It also helps to put facts over fears and to *keep on working.* As you exercise, tell yourself this:

- Exercise strengthens my muscles.
- Exercise relaxes me.
- Exercise improves my circulation.
- Exercise is good for me.

There will be days when you do not feel like doing the exercises. Remember, it's only a feeling. Do them anyway, and you'll find that you become more enthusiastic. *Doing* has a power of its own.

The bottom line is that it's important to make this routine a part of your life. If you stop doing it, you will lose your gains rather quickly.

Even with the best of intentions, however, you may stop for a while, since people are not perfect. If you experience this form of setback, don't blame yourself. Just get going again as soon as you can.

When you are able to work on *all* of the exercises without significant discomfort for two to four weeks, you can add the following three exercises to your routine:

EXERCISE #11:
Side Bending from a Chair

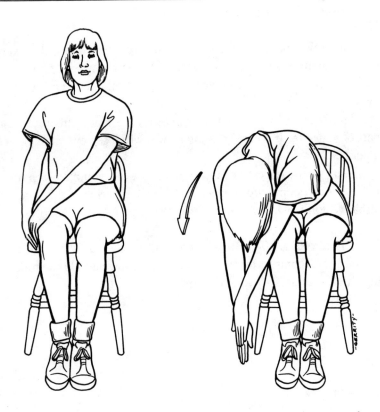

Sit forward on a straight, armless chair with your legs together, arms resting comfortably on your thighs.

1. Letting your arms drop to the right, bend down to your right. Go down only as far as you feel comfortable.

2. Slowly straighten your back and return to a sitting position, sliding your hands across your lap to the left.

3. Letting your arms drop to the left, bend down to your left.

4. Slowly straighten your back and return to a sitting position, sliding your hands across your lap to the right.

5. Repeat the entire exercise two times.

EXERCISE #12:
Hamstring/Calf Stretch

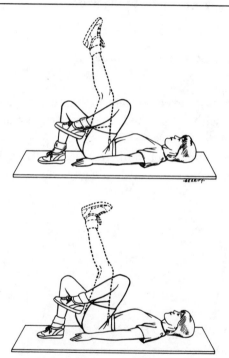

Lie on your back with your arms at your sides, feet on the floor, knees bent and slightly apart.

1. Bring right knee toward right shoulder, then straighten leg up toward the ceiling, as straight as you can, *pointing toe upward.*

2. Slowly lower right leg to the floor.

3. Slide right leg back to knee bent position.

4. Repeat steps 1, 2, and 3, bringing left knee to left shoulder, and so on.

5. Bring right knee to right shoulder, then straighten leg up toward the ceiling, this time *flexing the foot*—that is, keeping the sole facing the ceiling.

6. Slowly lower right leg to the floor.

7. Slide right leg back to the knee bent position.

8. Repeat steps 5, 6, and 7, bringing left knee to left shoulder, and so on.

9. Repeat entire exercise, alternating legs, for a total of eight more lifts, four with toe pointed and four with foot flexed.

Note: Pointing your toe upward stretches the hamstring muscles. Flexing your foot stretches both the hamstring and calf muscles.

EXERCISE #13:
Hamstring Stretch Standing

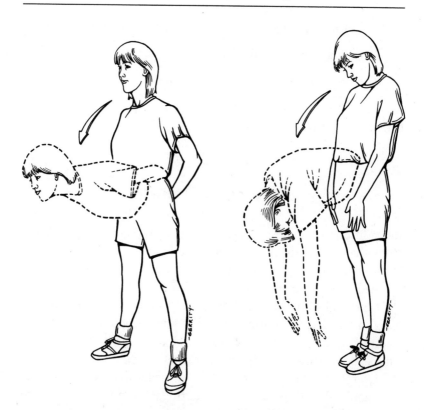

Stand with your feet slightly apart, hands behind your back and resting on the small of your back. Lock your knees.

1. While keeping your head up, bend forward at the waist as far as you can.

2. Return to an upright position, bending your knees as you do so.

3. Shake each leg individually to relax the muscles.

4. Bring legs together and lock your knees. Bring your arms around to the front. *Rest your chin on your chest.*

5. Drop your torso down to the floor as far as you comfortably can, letting your arms hang loose. Do not bounce or strain to touch the floor.

6. Return to upright position, bending your knees as you do so.

7. Shake each leg individually to relax the muscles.

8. Repeat the entire exercise two times.

Remember not to do more repeats of any exercises than are called for *until you are pain free.*

Walking for Strength
• • •

In addition to exercise, walking is an easy way to significantly strengthen the body and increase circulation. Make it a point to include walking in your exercise program. But here again, you must proceed in a gentle and gradual manner.

Start off by walking on a flat surface for only five to ten minutes each day, or less time, if need be. For some people with CPS, just walking up and down the block can be a big accomplishment. If this is all you can do at the moment, that's fine.

Even if you think you can walk for longer than ten minutes at first, don't. Plan to return to your starting point *before* you begin to feel uncomfortable. Gradually increase your time, a minute or so every few days. Be sure to wear laced-up, supportive walking shoes.

How you walk is important, too, as you know from your body awareness session. Avoid hitting the ground too hard. Instead, move your weight evenly from your heels to the balls of your feet. Maintain good posture and swing your arms easily. Look straight ahead and breathe in and out fluently. As you match your breathing to your stride, you'll find that walking also relaxes you.

Running, jogging, and sports other than swimming are *not* a good idea for CPS patients simply because they are too rough on the body. As for "working out," don't even think of using exercise machines until you have been pain free for at least one month and functioning confidently. Stick with walking and you'll find, as you will with the exercise routine, that even a little bit of physical work can go a long way toward alleviating your pain.

Another thing that can make a big difference is the way you look at the world and at the things that happen to you. As I mentioned earlier—pain is not only a perception, but a part of the *way* you perceive. By shifting your outlook and your response to events that trigger pain, you can significantly diminish pain. In the next chapter I'll teach you techniques for accomplishing this.

Coping with Pain-activating Triggers

S ince the eighteenth century, we have accepted that pain results when the nervous system responds to tissue damage. Injury sends a message to the spinal cord and then to the brain, signaling pain.

In recent decades, however, we have come to see that this understanding of pain is incomplete. We've noticed, for example, that soldiers in the heat of battle and athletes absorbed in a contest may not feel the pain of injuries until sometime afterward. We've also noticed that pain can persist after amputation, as if the missing arm or leg were still there (a phenomenon known as "phantom limb" pain). So tissue damage doesn't always produce immediate pain, nor is tissue damage necessary for pain to continue. Pain messages are sometimes delayed or seemingly inappropriate.

Clearly something besides the tissue damage itself must account for *when* and *how* we feel pain.

A revolutionary concept from two noted researchers, Patrick Wall, M.D., and Ronald Melzack, Ph.D., suggests an answer: There is a "gate control" mechanism in the brain, a series of chemical interactions, that controls the way pain messages are processed.

The gate seems to work this way: The damaged body part—a bad back, for example—sends a signal to the brain via the spinal cord. The brain *registers* a sensation, which is then altered by feelings, memories, and attitudes, and sends signals back to the spinal cord that *increase* or *decrease* the incoming stimulation, producing more or less pain.

So factors that are frequently thought to be nonphysical—emotions, memories, and the way we were brought up to think about pain and about life itself—can impact on the amount of pain we feel.

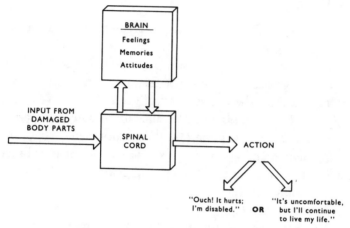

The implications of these discoveries for pain management are enormous. They mean that there are things we can do to keep the brain from increasing pain signals. By altering our thoughts and behaviors, we can discourage the strong, negative feelings that open the gate wider. By finding better ways of coping with situations that engender stress, we can encourage the gate to close as much as possible.

Now you can see why there is such a strong link between our minds and our bodies. The link doesn't mean that pain is "all in your head" and that you can just forget about it. It means that there is a connection between the way you think and act and the way pain signals are *processed* in your brain. You can't just "forget about" pain, but you can make behavioral choices that influence the chemistry controlling the "pain experience."

And when you combine these choices with the choices you have made to understand and strengthen your muscles, you can understand how powerful pain management can be. It works on both your physical and emotional selves, because these two entities are actually one.

Pain-activating Triggers
. . .

For people with CPS, stress is so closely related to increased pain that I call stressful events "pain-activating triggers" (PATs).

When you think of stress as a pain-activating trigger, you can see how dangerous it is. And you also understand why you must learn to cope with these triggers effectively.

As you know, coping can be difficult because pain-activating triggers seem to be everywhere in the environment. They are part of being human and also part of existing in our fast-paced society. I could fill several pages with these triggers, but let's list some you may commonly experience:

- You have too much to do and too little time.
- You get stuck in traffic jams and pushed and shoved on public transportation.
- Your boss yells at you.
- Your spouse or lover does things that annoy you.
- You've lost your job or taken on a new job.
- You're behind in meeting financial obligations.
- You're afraid you'll never be able to achieve the things you want to achieve.
- You have trouble balancing your work and your family.
- You worry about competition from co-workers.
- You worry about whether your children are engaging in harmful activities.

Those are just a few of the pain-activating triggers, or problems, that can set off pain in your head, shoulders, legs, back—you name it.

But notice the word *can*. All by themselves, these PATs are meaningless. Their power to influence the working of the pain gate depends upon the way you cope with them.

Coping is your control mechanism, your way of monitoring the gate. The importance of coping cannot be overestimated. And you have choices about the ways you cope.

To help you make the most of your coping abilities, let's first examine how you usually respond to pain-activating triggers and what choices you habitually make.

Think about the last major problem you faced. Try to remember as many details as possible. Then check off the ways you coped. Keep track of the letters next to the responses. I'll explain what the letters mean later.

• COPING QUIZ •

——I kept on going as if there weren't any problem. (A)

——I felt I had to solve the problem immediately. (I)

——I developed a few solutions that I thought might work. (PO)

——I felt angry at myself for getting into such a mess. (B)

——I relied on food, alcohol, cigarettes, or drugs to make myself feel better. (A)

——I tried not to act without thinking, even though I was experiencing strong emotions. (PO)

——I asked a person I have confidence in for some advice. (SS)

——I imagined myself getting revenge on the people who were causing the problem. (W)

——I felt bad because I had caused the problem. (B)

——I changed some of the ways I was acting so that I could solve the problem better. (PO)

——I kept the problem to myself. (A)

——I instinctively did whatever came into my head. (I)

——I tried not to do anything that would cut off avenues of communication. (PO)

——I wished that I was one of those people who know how to solve problems. (W)

____I stayed in bed a lot. (A)

____I realized it would take time to solve the problem, so I dealt with it one day at a time. (PO)

____I was mad as hell at the people who caused the problem. (A)

____I compromised so that even if I didn't get everything I wanted, I got some of what I wanted. (PO)

____I talked with someone I trust about the problem because I needed a sympathetic ear. (SS)

____I realized that I was feeling anxious and confused, but I didn't let that interfere with seeking a solution. (PO)

____I called myself a dope and other names for getting stuck with the problem. (B)

____I had to solve the problem right away, and when I couldn't, I wanted to stop trying. (I)

____I fantasized that I had enough power or money to solve the problem without doing anything. (W)

____I felt that I became a stronger person as a result of handling the problem. (PO)

Look at the responses you checked off, and the letters next to them, and let's discuss what those letters indicate about your coping strategies.

A stands for *avoidance*, the belief that running away will make the problem go away. It won't. Some avoidance behaviors, such as eating and drinking too much or turning to drugs, may bring the momentary comfort you crave. But they create major problems of their own. And they don't solve the problem at hand.

B stands for *blaming* yourself, a strategy that makes you feel lousy and doesn't touch the problem at all. Unless you enjoy diminishing your self-esteem, you can chalk this one up to wasted energy.

I stands for acting *impatiently* and emotionally. This strategy blows the situation out of the water more often than it solves the problem. True, you may get a temporary high from releasing your emotions, but that high is almost certainly followed by a crash.

W stands for *wishing*, fantasizing, and imagining the problem away. When you do this, you engage in another form of avoidance, because wishing is so absorbing that it's likely to keep you from coping with the problem at all.

You can see why avoiding, blaming yourself, being impatient, and wishing are not the coping strategies to choose. These measures heighten your emotions, increase your anxiety, and thereby also increase your receptivity to pain.

If you checked off *any* of them, watch out for these coping responses in the future.

Concentrate on the coping strategies indicated by the letters PO and SS. These are the strategies that are best for you.

PO stands for being *problem-oriented,* the most effective and meaningful way to cope. When you are problem-oriented, you do these things:

- You focus on the problem, not on your emotional reaction to it. You accept your feelings, but you don't let them drive you.
- You develop a plan of action that includes several alternative ways of solving the problem.
- You patiently keep trying, no matter how long it takes to reach a solution.
- You accept feelings of uncertainty and discomfort while working on the solution.
- You are willing to change things about yourself if this will help you reach a solution.
- You get satisfaction out of achieving a solution that is less than perfect.
- You view problem solving as an opportunity for personal growth.

The bottom line is that when you are problem-oriented, you cope. When you use such strategies as avoiding, blaming yourself, acting impatiently, and wishing, you fail to cope. *And disabling pain is associated with failed coping mechanisms.* This is why you, as a CPS sufferer, have to do everything you can to develop appropriate coping skills.

The letters SS stand for another appropriate skill, *seeking sup-*

port from others. All of us need to share problems by talking with people we trust. Their advice and empathy can help us solve problems better, although they cannot, of course, do the work for us. Connectedness encourages solutions and diminishes disabling pain.

Looking at Life the Way It Is
. . .

Why do some people choose coping strategies that influence the pain gate positively and other people do the opposite? The reason is that we select our strategies according to the way we *think* about the world. If we think in a way that leads us to cope poorly, we're stuck. So we have to examine our thinking before we can change our coping styles.

When I first introduced you to this program, I suggested that you evaluate yourself for thoughts that provoke pain. I hope you've become aware of them, because we're going to come down hard on some of those thoughts now.

Among the most harmful thoughts a person can have are the ones that focus on the word *should*.

- My husband *should* show more sympathy for me.
- My pain *should* go away.
- My boss *should* appreciate my work more.
- My doctors *should* cure me.

Other pain-provoking thoughts are the "I can't" statements:

- I *can't stand* this pain.
- I *can't stand* exercising.
- I *can't stand* being with people.
- I *can't stand* reading this book.

"Should" thoughts reveal the way we want other people or life itself to be. When things don't happen the way they "should," we get angry. "I can't" is really another way of saying "I won't" to anything new. So when events demand that we change the way we think and act, we find that we're immobilized.

"Should" and "I can't" thoughts also put blinders on us. With them we are not able to see reality. Walter Matweychuk, Ph.D., a dynamic psychologist who teaches this subject in my program, explains to patients that reality goes like this: We live in an imperfect world. Life is difficult and full of unsettling events. There are no easy solutions to life's problems. A lot of what happens to us is beyond our control. For all the effort we put in, there is no guarantee of success. We are not entitled to anything.

"Folks," Dr. Matweychuk says, "that's all there is. This is what we have to live with."

When we demand that life, we, or other people be as we want them to be, we compound the problems of pain. When we demand that we be rewarded for our efforts in life or relieved of our suffering, we compound the problems of pain. Conversely, when we accept life as it is and extract what satisfaction we can from its limitations, we decrease our perception of pain.

Now let's see how all of this applies to those pain-activating triggers a person with CPS might experience any day.

When he entered my program, Henry Carlson, the former construction worker I told you about at the beginning of this book, was in so much discomfort that he couldn't bend over to put on his shoes. His wife had to perform this task for him.

Although he politely thanked his wife for her assistance, inwardly Henry seethed. He hated feeling helpless and dependent. It diminished his self-image.

"I'm a person who can't even put on his shoes," Henry told me.

Every time Henry's wife helped him, Henry felt the pain in his neck and shoulders—the areas where he generally felt the most discomfort—increase significantly. After I explained the gate control theory, Henry could see that there was a connection between the anger he felt and the heightened pain.

I told Henry that the sequence went like this:

1. He needed help with his shoes.

2. He had certain thoughts about needing help.

3. The thoughts led to feelings of anger.

4. The anger was translated into muscle contractions, which increased pain in an already painful area.

PAT → thoughts → feelings → muscle contractions

We're not used to being aware of the thoughts that provoke our emotional responses, so it took Henry some time to see what I was getting at. Then he came up with what went through his mind whenever his wife assisted him: "I *should* be able to put on my shoes myself. I *shouldn't* need anyone's help."

It was the "should" thoughts that were provoking Henry's anger, not the circumstance of needing help with his shoes.

The fact that thoughts come between pain-activating triggers and our feelings gives us tremendous flexibility. We can alter our thoughts and, thereby, alter the intensity of our feelings. We can replace dogmatic "should" thinking with preferential thinking: "I would prefer things to happen in a certain way, but if they don't, I can live with it."

Let's see how Henry Carlson's scenario might proceed when he learns to think preferentially.

1. Henry's wife puts on his shoes.

2. Henry thinks, I would prefer not to need help with my shoes. *But I do.* So that's the way it is now. I hope it won't always be this way. But if it is, I can live with it.

3. Henry feels saddened by his situation but not angry. He does not experience an increase in pain.

4. Henry is also able to feel gratitude toward his wife, and he tells her, "Thank you, honey. I love you."

The point is that preferential thinking prevents a person from reacting to events with strong, negative emotions. It's like lowering a "feelings thermometer." And when you replace volatile emotions like anger, depression, and devastation with less volatile ones like annoyance, sadness, and disappointment, you decrease the signal of pain. You also make room for positive feelings and for connecting to those around you in a rewarding way.

Lowering volatile emotions has other advantages, too, as you can see if you think about just a few of the things such emotions do to you:

- They make you anxious.
- They make it difficult to concentrate.
- They make it difficult to have fun.
- They drive friends and family away from you.
- They drive you away from yourself.

Preferential thinking can help you avoid these pitfalls.

And there's another big plus: By *tuning in to reality, preferential thinking allows you to cope with pain-activating triggers in a problem-oriented manner.*

Some people seem to think preferentially naturally. Others have to work at it.

For these people—and it's most of us, I think—the tendency is to try to change a pain-activating trigger rather than the thoughts. Hitting out at the trigger engages negative emotions, and when that happens we usually don't act in our own best interests.

Take the case of one of my patients, Sandra Chamberlain.

Sandra had a boss who put a great deal of pressure on her. Every time he dumped an extra pile of papers on her desk at five o'clock, she thought, He's impossible. He *shouldn't* be behaving this way. Any decent person would have more consideration. And he knows about my lower back problems, too. Needless to say, when this happened Sandra experienced shooting pains in her back.

One day Sandra had enough. She quit her job, convinced she

was doing it because of the way her boss acted. She felt great at first, but it wasn't long before she realized that there were many things about her job that she liked. Now she was deprived of those satisfactions, not to mention her income. Her elation quickly turned to regret.

When Sandra joined my program, she learned that she had quit not because of her boss's behavior, but because of the "should" thoughts it evoked in her.

Sandra realized that thinking preferentially would have made her less angry. For example: I wish my boss wouldn't act as if he didn't give a damn about me. Perhaps he hasn't noticed how distraught that makes me. But I have to remember that people do what they want, not what I want. So I'll work on the aspects of this situation that I *can* control." Then Sandra could have asked her boss to prioritize which items had to be done that evening and which could be left for the next day.

Acting in this fashion would have downgraded Sandra's feelings from anger to annoyance. And annoyance doesn't make anyone walk out the door.

Sandra's relationship with her boss was a pain-activating trigger. She needed not to let him get to her so much and to be clear about what her needs were. But she couldn't do these things as long as she was thinking in terms of "should."

That's why, as Walter Matweychuk points out, it's best to work on our thoughts *before* we work on the pain-activating trigger. Then we're better equipped to cope with the trigger.

PAT → dogmatic thinking → change to preferential thinking → tone down emotions → solve problem posed by PAT

"Should" thinking can do more than keep you from coping. It can actually foster attitudes that drive you deeper into pain.

For example, let's imagine that one morning you wake up with more pain than you had the day before. You think: What did I do to deserve this? I've always been such a good person. Life *should* be more fair.

You feel yourself getting depressed and angry. The anger heightens your pain, leading to more depression. You decide to stay in bed and skip your exercise routine. You may even cancel a luncheon appointment. You allow pain to take over your day. Pain-button thinking has made your pain worse and your life miserable.

But if you practice thinking preferentially, you can hold this sort of dysfunction off at the pass. You can think, Okay, I'm feeling more pain. I wish there would be less pain every day. But I know it doesn't work that way. There will be ups and downs. I'll keep doing my exercises, and I hope I'll feel better tomorrow.

By thinking preferentially, you can keep up your determination. You can draw the line on anger and depression.

Taking Your Emotional Temperature
• • •

Like your levels of pain, the way you think and the emotions generated by your thinking vary throughout the day.

At one o'clock in the afternoon, after a relatively pain-free morning, it's easier to respond to a pain-activating event with annoyance rather than anger. At eight o'clock at night, after a day full of PATs, you're more likely to respond to yet another one with anger.

Just as you tracked your daily pain levels using the visual analog scales, it's a good idea to track your emotional levels, too. That way you can discover when you're most vulnerable to rigid thinking.

For a day or two, take your emotional pulse every few hours or so. On a piece of paper, sketch the chart shown on page 102. Leave plenty of room to jot down those emotions you are aware of, particularly the ones you experience in response to pain-activating triggers.

TIME	EMOTIONS
A.M.	
6	
7	
8	
9	
10	
11	
12	
P.M.	
1	
2	
3	
4	
5	
6	
7	
8	
9	
10	
11	

Looking at the chart, you'll be able to see how many feelings
—joy, anger, annoyance, depression, pleasure, and so forth—you

may experience in the course of a day. Pay particular attention to the powerful negative emotions, and try to remember the thoughts you were having when you experienced them. Most likely you'll remember that a few "should" thoughts were going through your mind. Resolve to substitute preferential thinking for rigid thinking whenever you can. This isn't easy. It takes practice. It takes time. But, believe me, it can work.

Remember that pain-activating triggers only give you an opportunity to get upset. But you don't have to bite. You don't have to make yourself hurt more. *You have a choice.*

Another way to diminish your pain is to increase your tolerance for discomfort. Right now you're probably thinking: *What? He's saying I should allow myself to feel more uncomfortable?*

No. *Tolerating* discomfort and *feeling* uncomfortable are not the same. In fact, they are mutually exclusive. When you learn to tolerate discomfort, the discomfort lessens, because it becomes defused.

Generally, people with chronic pain syndrome have low discomfort tolerance. Pain makes them tense, irritable, and extremely sensitive to pain-activating triggers. They are caught in a cycle of pain, strong emotions, and more pain, so no wonder they become less tolerant of just about everything.

You can break the cycle at any point by using a number of coping techniques. One, for example, is body awareness, which allows you to move in a way that circumvents pain. Another is exercise, which relaxes and strengthens the weakened muscles that make you susceptible to pain. A third, preferential thinking, tones down the emotions that trigger pain.

Learning to tolerate discomfort is another useful technique. You do this simply by being aware that you *can* do it.

The key is to work at banishing the "I can't" statements, which are actually another form of rigid thinking. As I said earlier, probably no other phrase more effectively keeps people with CPS from getting better than "I can't." Once you think, I can't, you stop doing everything: body awareness movements, exercises, thinking preferentially, and so on. "I can't" is like a stop sign at a railroad crossing. You have to tear it down and replace it with this:

I can stand the discomfort of doing whatever I have to do to make my life better.

Granted, it's a big sign—but you need it.

How do you erect such a sign in your life? Think about the things you need to do to manage your pain. Then think about the rewards you will gain when you do those things. Realize that you *can* stand the discomfort for the sake of the rewards.

Some people find it helpful to write down what they can stand. They post these statements where they can see them easily, on the refrigerator, for example, or on the bathroom mirror.

Here are some statements that Walter Matweychuk suggests you might come up with:

- *I can stand* the discomfort of feeling sore when I first begin to exercise because I know that exercise will help relieve my pain.
- *I can stand* the discomfort of dieting because being thinner will make me healthier.
- *I can stand the discomfort* of learning to think positively because I know that my life will be happier when I give up blaming and catastrophizing.
- *I can stand the discomfort* of getting better gradually rather than all at once, because I know that is the only real way to get better.
- *I can stand the discomfort* of making compromises because I know that doing so will allow me to solve problems.

You can probably add several of your own. The point is to select the "I can" statements that are most important to you and concentrate on them.

Bear in mind that tolerance for discomfort develops *gradually* and requires working on *consistently*. It's hard stuff, so don't be disappointed if you fail sometimes. The important thing is to keep at it.

As your tolerance for discomfort increases, and you learn to think preferentially, you'll find yourself coping better with pain-activating triggers and with pain itself. You will be closer to your goal of managing your pain. And you will feel better about yourself, too.

Detaching Yourself from Pain

I magine a hot-air balloon tied to the earth by mooring lines. Now imagine that the lines begin to loosen, one by one, and the balloon floats free of its moorings. Just as that balloon can detach itself from the earth, you can detach yourself from pain.

Right now, though, rather than detaching from pain, you have detached from almost *everything else*. But thanks to the complicated nature of the brain itself, you can detach from pain. The brain is bombarded by thousands of signals each minute but can attend to just so many of them, as attested to by the gate control theory. When you use certain techniques, and observe certain principles, the brain is encouraged to overlook the pain signals.

A primary way to detach is through relaxation. I don't mean for you to relax by getting into a hot tub, though that can be useful, too. I am talking about the sort of relaxation process that alters your physiology and induces a quieter, more pain-free state.

This process can be practiced and mastered. You've mastered some of it already by learning diaphragmatic breathing—breathing so that your belly expands while your chest remains still. This, as you probably noticed, gives you a distinctly relaxed feeling.

In this exercise, diaphragmatic breathing, visual imaging (picturing yourself in a pleasant place or circumstance), and autosuggestion (telling yourself positive things through the subconscious mind) work together to loosen your connection to pain.

Before you begin, read all of the instructions carefully and commit them to memory as well as you can. It's even better if someone can read the instructions to you, in a calm, quiet voice, as you try them the first few times.

The Relaxation Practice
. . .

It's best to do this while seated, but if you find extended sitting painful, you can stand up or lie down. (Just try not to fall asleep.)

Select a chair that allows your feet to rest on the ground comfortably. Sit in an easy position, with arms and legs uncrossed and hands resting on your knees. Let your muscles let go as much as possible.

Close your eyes and begin to breathe slowly and deeply into your belly. Keep your chest still. Feel your belly inflate as you breathe in and deflate as you breathe out.

Now, start to count slowly, one—two—three as you inhale and three—two—one as you exhale. Work to match your breathing to the counting. Keep your chest relatively still. Each time you breathe out, try to relax a little more and then still more.

Breathe in and out in this manner for a minute or so. Then, as you continue to breathe slowly and easily, start to fill your mind with the details of a pleasant place. Perhaps it's a white sandy beach, a sunlit forest, or a flower-filled garden, wherever you think you'd be happy, comfortable, and at ease. Let yourself *be* in this place. Notice its colors, sounds, textures, and temperature.

Stay in the comfortable place, breathing in and out gently. With each breath, you may notice that your muscles are becoming less tight.

Let your mind's eye sweep over your body from head to toe, looking for remaining muscular tightness. Check your face, eyes, jaw, neck, shoulders, upper arms, forearms, hands, upper back, lower back, buttocks, thighs, calves, and feet. *Allow* your muscles to feel looser. *Allow* yourself to fall further into a relaxed state.

Continue to be aware of your breathing and the comfortable place you have created:

As you breathe, slowly repeat each of the following lines to yourself several times:

"My right arm is beginning to feel heavy."
"My right arm is feeling heavy."
"My right arm is feeling quite heavy."
"My left arm is beginning to feel heavy."
"My left arm is feeling heavy."
"My left arm is feeling quite heavy."
"My arms are feeling quite heavy."
"My shoulders are beginning to feel heavy."
"My shoulders are feeling heavy."
"My shoulders are feeling quite heavy."
"My right leg is beginning to feel heavy."
"My right leg is feeling heavy."
"My right leg is feeling quite heavy."
"My left leg is beginning to feel heavy."
"My left leg is feeling heavy."
"My left leg is feeling quite heavy."
"My arms, legs, and shoulders are feeling quite heavy."

Be still for a little moment or two. Let go of all muscle tension. You'll probably feel yourself sinking deeper into your comfortable place.

Now say these lines:

"My right arm is beginning to feel heavy and warm."
"My right arm is feeling heavy and warm."
"My right arm is feeling quite heavy and warm."
"My left arm is beginning to feel heavy and warm."
"My left arm is feeling heavy and warm."
"My left arm is feeling quite heavy and warm."
"My arms are feeling quite heavy and warm."
"My shoulders are beginning to feel heavy and warm."

"My shoulders are feeling heavy and warm."

"My shoulders are feeling quite heavy and warm."

"My right leg is beginning to feel heavy and warm."

"My right leg is feeling heavy and warm."

"My right leg is feeling quite heavy and warm."

"My left leg is beginning to feel heavy and warm."

"My left leg is feeling heavy and warm."

"My left leg is feeling quite heavy and warm."

"My arms, legs, and shoulders are feeling quite heavy and warm."

Focus your attention on the words as you say them to yourself. Continue with these lines:

"My breathing is beginning to feel calm and regular."

"My breathing is feeling calm and regular."

"My breathing is feeling quite calm and regular."

"My heartbeat is beginning to feel calm and regular."

"My heartbeat is feeling calm and regular."

"My heartbeat is feeling quite calm and regular."

"My breathing and heartbeat are quite calm and regular."

"My shoulders, arms, and legs are feeling quite heavy and warm."

"My breathing and heartbeat are quite calm and regular."

You should notice yourself feeling heavier and entering a highly relaxed state. You may not be aware of anything but the sound of your own breathing. You may not feel any pain. Or your pain may seem to be far away from you and unimportant. *Allow yourself to enjoy being pain free or pain distant.*

To get yourself out of the relaxed state, slowly raise your right arm. Let it drop gently onto your knee. Then focus on your breathing, leaving the comfortable place behind. As you notice your breathing, you'll become more aware of your physical surroundings. When you're ready, without making any sudden movements—open your eyes.

Some people experience strong feelings of relaxation during their first practice. If that happened to you, try to remember the subtle differences between being relaxed and not being relaxed.

Commit them to memory. That way you'll know what you want to achieve when you practice relaxation.

If you didn't feel very relaxed, don't worry. Barrie Guise, Ph.D., the empathetic psychologist who works with my patients on relaxation, finds that most people need to do it a number of times before they begin to see significant effects. In fact, it takes about three or four months to master this technique totally.

But when you "get it," you really get it, as Dr. Guise says. Relaxation becomes automatic, and in what seems like a "moment" you will be able to call into play all of the physiological changes learned in the practice. You will then have yet another mechanism at your disposal for dealing with such pain-activating triggers as traffic jams, hassles with co-workers, and so forth. That's quite a payoff for a relatively small input of time.

If you choose to learn relaxation, plan to do the practice for fifteen minutes at least once a day, perferably early in the morning because it can get you ready for the day. The only time to avoid practicing is after a big meal, because then you will be competing with the activities of your digestive system.

How to Handle "Interfering" Thoughts

· · ·

When they first begin to practice relaxation, patients can experience thoughts and images that challenge their ability to concentrate. They may find themselves thinking about noises in the room or reviewing yesterday's shopping list. Or they may see disturbing images. One patient told me, for example, that she saw a building collapsing when she tried to relax.

The thing to remember about these intruders, Barrie Guise emphasizes, is that they are okay. Let them happen. You can have different thoughts, images, and sensations and *still* relax. You can think, My brain has thoughts. That's no surprise. I'm not going to try to push the thoughts away. I'm going to *allow* myself to have them, and then I'll *allow* myself to concentrate again.

Notice the emphasis on the word *allow*. I use it because relaxation is actually *passive concentration*. It's something that you let happen. You have to work at it, but you can't force it. *You must relax about relaxing.*

There's something else to be aware of when you first start to relax: you may notice an increase, rather than a decrease, in pain. There are several reasons for this. Scanning your body can make you aware of sore spots you didn't feel before. Very tight muscles may hurt as they start to relax. Or you may have an unconscious resistance to relaxing that makes you turn the process inside out. For example, one of my patients insisted that her hands got colder when she told herself they were getting warmer.

Some people experience unsettling emotions when they try to relax, and this may happen to you. Unconsciously you may have been using muscle tension to bottle up feelings. If you can let these feelings out, the muscles can relax and your pain decrease. If you feel a desire to cry, don't fight it. Try to trust your feelings and to be open to them. (I'll have more to say about feelings in a later chapter.)

There's no doubt that relaxation is powerful and effective. Be assured that your pain *will* diminish as you continue to practice. If you are a very tense person, you may have to practice more—but that only means you have a longer road to travel, not that you should give up.

After you have practiced the technique consistently, you'll find that the physiological steps become compressed and you can often achieve a relaxed state rather quickly, sometimes in a matter of moments.

Even when you reach this stage, Barrie Guise suggests, call up a relaxation response as often as you can during the day, whether or not you are in stressful situations. *Remember, the time to relax is before you have to relax.* Relax regularly, and you will be better prepared for pain-activating triggers when they occur.

Another rule is to start relaxing at the *first sign* of a pain-activating trigger, when you first get stuck in a traffic jam, for example, not when you realize it will go on for at least an hour.

To start relaxing before a pain-activating trigger makes you tense, you must be aware of your body's preliminary signals of stress, such as increased heartbeat, clammy hands, dizziness, anxious feelings—whatever applies to you. Keep these signals in mind, put relaxation skills into play, and you will be able to detach yourself from threats of increased pain before they become full blown.

Getting Away from It All
. . .

I want you to think back to the last time you were really absorbed in something, a joke someone was telling you, an interesting conversation with a friend, or a good movie. You'll probably recall that while you were involved in these events, you noticed your pain less or your pain may have disappeared altogether. Distractions of this sort can be very powerful. They can neutralize the experience of pain in the same way that anesthesia does. Distraction is another way of detaching.

But if you're like most chronic pain sufferers, you've been finding it increasingly difficult to get distracted. Pain seems to push everything else out of the way. *It* has become your major distraction. Now you need to work on letting life distract you from pain.

"I try, but I just can't seem to concentrate on anything else," patients frequently tell me. Although you may believe that, it isn't totally true. Distraction has the power to sneak up on people, even people in pain.

Here's an example: One day, in a group session, a patient told a story about how he had outwitted a shady used-car dealer. This man was a born raconteur, and his story was genuinely funny. By the time he'd finished, everyone in the room was convulsed with laughter.

When the room quieted down, Barrie Guise asked who could remember feeling any pain while laughing. No one could, even though two or three people had reported being severely uncomfortable just a few seconds before the storyteller began. My patients had not chosen to be distracted by this story. Yet somehow they'd *allowed* themselves to be distracted, and it worked.

Our availability to be distracted never leaves us, even though pain may cast a pall over it. But pain or no pain, we can take advantage of it. We can actively seek situations that have a good chance of absorbing us. We don't have to wait for a happy chance, like coming in contact with a skilled storyteller or having someone throw a surprise birthday party for us. *We can take control.*

It takes some doing, but we can

- socialize with friends.
- play games with our family.
- engage in old hobbies or start a new one.
- read about something that interests us.
- go to a play, movie, or sporting event.
- travel, even if we take only short day trips.

We can do these, and hundreds of other things, *while we are in pain.* After all, we're in pain anyway, so why not try to distract ourselves? If it works, we're ahead of the game. If it doesn't, we've lost nothing. Try it: it works.

One of my patients, Rosalind White, wanted to see if what I was saying was accurate. In spite of her pain, she got on a bus for the seashore. "I decided that I might as well have my pain in a pleasant setting," she told me. But toward the middle of the day, as she was looking at the ocean after a walk with a friend along the boardwalk and a visit to a nearby bird sanctuary, Rosalind noticed that her pain was gone. She couldn't help smiling to herself. By choosing to get absorbed in an interesting day, Rosalind had suc-ceeded in eliminating her pain.

Is Distraction Worth the Effort?
• • •

If you decide to distract yourself, as Rosalind did, the amount of pain relief you get may not be very great—at first.

"Oh, that distraction stuff lasts only for a little while," a patient once complained while reaching for a pill whose effects also lasted only a little while. No difference, right? Wrong.

Being able to distract yourself for short periods of time soon leads to being able to distract yourself for longer periods of time. Swallowing pills only leads to swallowing more pills.

Like every other technique in this book, distraction becomes more useful the more you use it. It's a question of practice, practice, practice—and of accepting the idea that the payoffs will start out small and grow gradually:

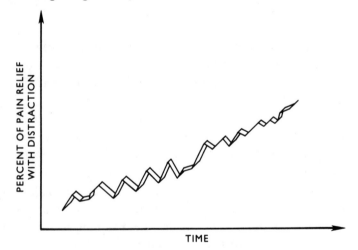

As you make more and more efforts to distract yourself, you'll find—as you will with relaxation—that you have developed a skill that works almost automatically.

When that happens, you can use distraction not only to get away from pain, but also to get your life back into balance. A sense of balance, like distraction, is a way of loosening the moorings to pain.

Balance is achieved when we put pleasure back into our lives, when we rescue those aspects of our humanity that have been stolen from us. Balance is a conscious attempt to combine what we *must* do with what we *enjoy* doing and with what *nourishes* us spiritually.

By now you're familiar enough with this program not to be surprised when I tell you that it takes work. For starters, you have to believe in it. Then you have to make an effort to structure your day to achieve it. I'll have more to say about this when we talk about time management. In the meantime it can help to think about these resolutions:

1. Every day, I will perform at least one task that I enjoy doing.

2. Every day, I will consciously enjoy the sensory pleasures of sight, sound, smell, touch, and taste.

3. Every day, I will enjoy the company of those I love.

4. Every day, I will be grateful for my family, friends, and co-workers.

5. Every day, I will make time to do a kindness for someone.

6. Every day, I will do something I enjoy doing all by myself.

Even though I used the word *enjoy* several times in the balance program, the key word for achieving balance is "gratitude." When you remember to be grateful for the things around you—nature, family, friends—and within you—talents, skills, feelings—you see the value of life in all of its variety. You want to be able to experience it and to enjoy it. You want to bolster your determination to leave pain behind.

How Acceptance Fosters Detachment
• • •

First off, let me say that I'm *not* asking you to accept your pain. What I am asking you to accept is that you are not the same person you were before you developed chronic pain syndrome. And, much as you will improve, you may never be exactly the same person again. This is normal. Every living thing changes. As we grow older, we lose some capacities but gain others. But whatever changes you have undergone, *you can still be the best that you can be now.*

This is a concept that many CPS sufferers find difficult. They want to be the way they were before—and quickly. Sometimes a patient will say, "If I can't do everything the way I used to, it's not worth doing anything at all." But if you think like that, you *won't* do anything at all, and your pain will increase. The truth is that to feel less pain, you need to accept some aspects of your new situation.

Remember my patient, Henry Carlson, who found it difficult to accept his wife's help in putting on his shoes? That was just one of the many changes Henry had experienced as a result of his injury. Let's look at a few of them:

OLD HENRY	NEW HENRY
Held down a good-paying job	Receives workers' compensation
Did most of the household repairs	Needs help putting on his shoes
Organized family events	Feels too uncomfortable to participate in family events
Was an active basketball player	Can't play basketball
Had frequent sexual relations	The less said the better (thinks this will never change)

You probably could make a similar list. *The changes you have experienced as a result of your pain—the differences between the old and new you—represent losses for which you must mourn if you are to decrease your pain.*

Some people do this grieving naturally. Others, I have found, need to give themselves permission. They have to allow themselves to feel sad rather than anxious or angry. One of my patients, who was angry most of the time, was finally able to say, "I miss the simple things I used to do, like taking a walk." After saying that, he burst into tears. Soon he was able to discuss other losses, and a short time later his mood became more accepting.

Think about the losses you may have experienced. Allow yourself to cry for them, if necessary. Once the mourning is behind you, it's possible to move on to establishing yet another you: *a person whose life has changed but who compensates for losing some things by maximizing others.*

There are several steps toward achieving this type of acceptance:

Step One. Understand that no matter where you are right now, you are a good and valuable person. Banish those thoughts about what you "should" be able to do physically in order to feel good about yourself. "Should" thinking, as you have already seen, has little to do with the real world. Allow your self-acceptance to be unconditional. *Unconditional self-acceptance works to detach you from the suffering that frequently accompanies persistent pain.*

Step Two. Understand that while you cannot do everything you used to do, there are many things you can do. *You have to be flexible.* For example, Henry Carlson had to give up basketball, but with his wife's help he was able to do a little cross-country skiing. Another patient, who was unable to continue his work as a carpenter, took up wood carving. If you can accept not having *exactly* what you used to want, you'll find that there are quite a few things you can still do. *You can create a full life, even if it's not the way you thought it would be.*

Step Three. Understand that acceptance comes from trusting life and in abandoning our own need to change what cannot be changed. The great French novelist Marcel Proust put it this way: "We do not succeed in changing things according to our desire, but gradually our desire changes. The situation that we hoped to change because it was intolerable becomes unimportant. We have not managed to surmount the obstacle, as we were absolutely determined to do, but life has taken us around it, led us past it, and then if we turn around to gaze at the remote past, we can barely catch sight of it, so imperceptible has it become."

Try to keep the picture in mind of an obstacle becoming imperceptible. See how this relates to the picture I painted earlier of the balloon floating away from the earth. Both are detachment images. And like that balloon, you can break free of your old self-image and replace it with a new, but no less worthwhile, self-image.

Don't Think of Pain as Punishment
• • •

There's yet another detachment mechanism, and it has to do with eliminating what I call the pain anticipation response.

Even when they don't feel pain, many people with CPS are constantly tense in anticipation of its return. They may even feel uneasy if the pain *doesn't* show up, because it means they will be "paid back" later. They act as if pain were a mean person instead of a process.

I hear remarks like "The pain is getting back at me for the good time I had yesterday" or "The pain is really letting me have it for those eight hours of sleep."

Every time we anticipate pain, and every time we personify it in this way, we make it stronger. "Render unto Caesar the things that are Caesar's," says the Bible. But all too often we pay tribute to pain instead of putting it in its proper place.

This kind of behavior may have its roots in childhood, when our parents punished us for doing something wrong. The punishment involved physical or emotional pain, so we started to associate pain with having done something wrong. Now, when we experience pain, we may think: What did I do to deserve this? Why am I being punished? Or a phrase many of us heard as children—"I'll really give you something to cry about"—may flash through our minds. These memories validate pain as punishment.

When such memories influence adult behavior, they constitute "pain-button thinking" of a very high order.

You must make an effort to detach from this thinking. The next time you catch yourself "expecting" pain, ask yourself, Why do I feel this way? Most likely you'll find it's because you believe pain has some power over you. The detachment mechanism is actively to *disbelieve*.

Tell yourself this:

- I do not have to anticipate pain. When I am free of pain, I can behave as though it does not have to come back.
- If pain does return, I do not have to think that it is punishing me. Instead I can practice the relaxation techniques that will lessen the pain.
- I do not have to think that pain has power over me. It does not.

You need to work very hard on these thoughts to readjust your perspective. Just as you can use relaxation to detach yourself from pain, you can use readjustments in your thinking, too.

So there are many ways to loosen your moorings to pain. Choose those that seem most effective for you. Work on them consistently. And you will find that, like that balloon, you have the capacity to float away from pain.

Why Painkillers Can Be a Trap

There's bad news and good news about chronic pain and drugs. The bad news is that the so-called painkilling drugs—those that work directly on the pain pathways —can frequently make you feel worse. The good news—and it's pretty ironic, too—is that some drugs that were not even developed to treat pain can be your best bet for relief.

So even though I'm going to tell you why you have to re-evaluate your use of painkillers, keep in mind that there are other drugs out there that can be substituted for them if necessary. Later on I'll explain how these "good news" drugs work. For a start, though, let's face the truth about painkillers.

Painkillers: One Size Doesn't Fit All
• • •

Acute pain and chronic pain, as you know, are quite different. Yet both are treated with the same types of drugs, painkillers. Painkillers are a boon to someone suffering from acute pain—as with terminal cancer, for example—but they can create big problems for someone like you who has probably been using them over long periods of time. *Constant use makes these drugs dangerous, even if they are the kind you can buy over the counter.*

If you take painkillers regularly, you are going to have to decide whether to continue your current level of use, reduce it, or stop all together. As you will see, there are many reasons to consider the latter two courses.

Bear that in mind as we review the three categories of pain-killers most commonly prescribed for chronic pain:

❑ *Nonsteroidal anti-inflammatory drugs (NSAIDs).* These drugs work, in part, by reducing the inflammation that may be a cause of pain. They include aspirin, buffered aspirin (Alka-Seltzer, Bufferin), and such aspirinlike drugs as ibuprofen (Advil, Motrin, Nuprin), Clinoril, Dolobid, and Voltaren.

❑ *Acetaminophen* (Tylenol) provides symptomatic relief from pain but does not reduce inflammation and is, therefore, not a true NSAID. It is frequently prescribed for people who cannot tolerate aspirin.

❑ *Opioid analgesics.* These drugs contain natural or synthetic opiates and act on the spinal cord and brain stem to produce their analgesic effect. Among the commonly prescribed opioids are co-deine and the following combination drugs that also contain an NSAID or Tylenol: aspirin with codeine, Tylenol with codeine, Darvon compound, Darvocet, Percocet, and Percodan.

All of these drugs may provide some pain relief, but they all have a substantial down side. When it comes to drugs, there is no free lunch.

For example, let's consider the first category, the NSAIDs, which many patients consider "innocuous." Used over long periods of time, these drugs can have serious gastric side effects (which is why they should never be taken on an empty stomach). Long-term use of NSAIDs can result in ulcers and stomach bleeds. And since it is possible to have an ulcer without being aware of it, you could develop a serious bleed from these "harmless" drugs.

There's another caution, too. Aspirin and aspirinlike medications can cause "rebound pain," pain that stems from the drugs themselves. I had one patient who took aspirin every day for fifty years for headaches. The headaches didn't stop until he *stopped* taking the aspirin.

Acetaminophen (Tylenol), the second category, doesn't cause stomach problems—that's one of its major attributes—but excessive use can result in liver and kidney damage.

Although these adverse side effects are not common, they can occur when people with chronic pain don't keep track of how long they've been taking a nonprescription drug or how much of it they use. And their tendency is to use more of a drug than they realize.

The NSAIDs and Tylenol have a *ceiling level* for effectiveness. If you go above that level, you do not experience more relief, but you do experience more serious side effects.

It's advisable to keep the following don'ts posted near your medicine cabinet:

- *Don't* take more of any drug than your physician has prescribed or the bottle says is safe.
- *Don't* take more than one of the same category of drug—two NSAIDs, for example. Mixing in this manner makes each drug less effective and more poisonous to your body.
- *Don't* mix NSAIDs and Tylenol.
- *Don't* use any drug unless you are sure that it is helping you.

The last point sounds pretty obvious, but you can get so used to a painkilling drug regimen that you stop evaluating its effectiveness. You cannot afford to be haphazard, however, because every drug has its price in side effects. *A painkiller that isn't helping you can be harming you,* and therefore you should discuss with your physician any medication you are taking routinely.

The Opioid Trap

· · ·

Opioids are a boon for people in acute pain, such as postsurgical pain, and for that small percentage of chronic pain patients with problems not treatable by the means detailed in this book. More than 95 perecent of people with CPS, however, do better not taking opioids over the long term, I believe. These drugs can produce serious side effects, including constipation, depression, drug tolerance, and drug dependency.

Tolerance means that your body becomes resistant to the opioid's effectiveness and you need higher and higher doses to obtain the same level of relief. (A first sign, for example, is when a pill that used to work for four hours now works only for three.) Dependency means that your body needs the drug, and if you stop taking it, you may experience withdrawal symptoms. If you continue to take the opioid, you may find that you can accomplish less and less, even though you feel your pain is diminished.

Every day I see patients who can't be roused out of their stupors or who fall asleep intermittently, often right in the middle of a group discussion. "Are you with me?" I ask these people, and quite often they are too drugged to answer.

In short, opioid use can be a pit. As it reduces your pain, it may also reduce your ability to function.

One patient I remember in particular was Thomas Ivans, a young man who insisted that painkillers were helping him, even though he was too wiped out to get out of his chair, much less think about doing some exercises. His fiancée was talking about leaving him. (In fact, it was she who had insisted that he join my program.) Tom had long since left his job. His existence had come down to pill taking and sleeping. Yet he thought this was what he had to expect.

It isn't. When painkillers are killing your life, rather than making it better, you are paying too high a price for them.

Since you've committed yourself to being tougher with yourself —that's one of the things this program is all about—you need to be completely honest with yourself about your use of painkillers. While looking your pill bottles straight in the face, ask yourself these questions:

1. Do I have trouble concentrating?

2. Do I suffer frequent lapses of memory?

3. Do I find it difficult to perform the simplest tasks?

4. Do I have mood swings?

5. Do I "drop out" of conversations?

6. Am I tired all the time?

The more yes answers you come up with, the more impaired you probably are.

If you want to function better, the tradeoff is to use lesser amounts of these drugs or none of them at all.

The choice is yours. But the fact that you decided to participate in this program—which focuses so strongly on functioning—probably indicates that you are willing to reduce your use of painkillers.

Even so, I know it can sometimes be difficult to go forward. You're tired of painkillers, yet you worry about the pain you *think* you'll feel if you stop taking them. This combination of weariness and fear is common to chronic pain sufferers.

At some point, however, the weariness has to overcome the fear. You can tip the balance by remembering that there are other drugs you can turn to, if necessary—drugs I'll tell you about in a little while. You can also let your weariness work for you by telling yourself this:

- I'm tired of feeling drugged all the time.
- I'm tired of needing that next pill.
- I'm tired of being afraid to be *without* painkillers.
- I'm going to make a switch: I'm going to believe that functioning well is more important than painkillers.

Are You Ready to Cut Back?
· · ·

Here comes that word *gradually* again. The way to break free of drugs is to decrease the amounts you use *in stages,* under your doctor's supervision. Never, never stop using a drug abruptly.

But don't even think about reducing painkiller usage until you have experienced success with other aspects of this program. If you start to cut back too soon, you will almost certainly fail. Wait until you notice some improvement from body awareness, the exercises, coping techniques, relaxation techniques, or more positive ways of thinking. You won't be ready to cut back until you have some sense of mastery over your pain by other means.

The only exception to this rule is if you are so impaired that you can't even work on the other parts of this program without reducing opioid drug use, or the use of other habit-forming drugs such as tranquilizers and sedatives. Tom Ivans, the young man who slept most of the time, wouldn't even have been able to follow the simplest instructions had he continued his opioid level, so I started to cut it back.

Most people, however, should hold back on reducing drugs for a while. You don't need to wait until all of the nondrug techniques are working, or until they are working perfectly (they never will be), but you do need to wait until you have realized that other methods of fighting pain can help you. This realization will help you fight your dependence on drugs.

If you have been doing the exercises described earlier faithfully for some time, you are ready to evaluate whether you are ready for drug reduction. One way to do so is by keeping your "pain evaluation diary," with visual analog scales.

A visual analog scale, as you remember, is just a simple line that allows you to measure your pain. It looks like this:

NO PAIN ├─────────────────────────────┤ **MOST PAIN IMAGINABLE**

Your diary will consist of several scales for different times of the day:

TODAY'S DATE: _____

1. **Waking up** ├─────────────────────────┤

2. **Midmorning** ├─────────────────────────┤

3. **Midafternoon** ├─────────────────────────┤

4. **Dinnertime** ├─────────────────────────┤

5. **Bedtime** ├─────────────────────────┤

On each scale, at about the times indicated, make a mark where you feel your pain level to be. Compare it with the scales you made when you began this program. You should notice that you are experiencing lower levels of pain.

The levels may be *significantly* lower or *somewhat* lower. Keep in mind, though, that small degrees of improvement can count for a lot. Small amounts become large amounts in time.

You might also want to make another check of your motivation level, which was first discussed when you began this program. Has that level gone up? Have you established goals for what you want to do when your pain is better?

If you have started making concrete plans for the future, if you have begun to feel more enthusiastic about life itself, this program is having an effect. You are ready to proceed with the brave step of opioid drug reduction.

Getting Off Painkillers
· · ·

Before getting off painkillers, the first thing you must do is discuss the matter with your physician. Most likely he or she will support your efforts to cut back, since doctors are not happy about providing large amounts of opioid analgesics, sedatives, or tranquilizers.

Most likely, too, if you are taking more than one drug, you'll be advised to reduce only one at a time. This makes the process safer and the effect of each drug on your body easier to determine.

How does drug reduction work? *You need to take 20 percent less of the drug than you normally do for two days, then cut back by an additional 20 percent every two days thereafter.* For example, let's say that you are currently using three tablets of Tylenol with codeine every four hours (even though it's possible that only two tablets were prescribed). Your reduction regimen would look this:

Days one and two—take 2½ pills every four hours.
Days three and four—take 2 pills every four hours.
Days five and six—take 1½ pills every four hours.
Days seven and eight—take 1 pill every four hours.
Days nine and ten—take ½ pill every four hours.

By reducing in this graded manner, you would be free of the drug by day eleven.

At a measured pace, it's unusual to feel discomfort, and many people experience an increased sense of well-being. But if you've become highly dependent on a drug, you may undergo withdrawal symptoms, such as increased blood pressure, sweating, tremors, diarrhea, nausea, irritability, and sleeplessness. You may also notice a *temporary* increase in pain. If the drug you're reducing is an opioid, the increased pain should last only about three days. If the drug is a tranquilizer, it may last for up to a week, since it's even more difficult to break free of tranquilizers than it is opioids.

Another thing about opioids is that since they are mood-altering drugs, the pain you think you feel may not be pain at all but an increase in anxiety. That's why it's important to sort out your feelings and, if necessary, step up your use of techniques that reduce anxiety, such as exercise and relaxation. I will have more to say about anxiety in a later chapter on feelings.

Though most people do not find it particularly difficult to cut back on painkillers, if you think you might have trouble, prepare beforehand.

Be ready to rely on the pain management techniques you have learned thus far. When you feel like reaching for a pill, do one of the following:

- Practice a relaxation technique.
- Perform your exercises.
- Execute your body awareness movements.
- Go for a walk.
- Distract yourself in other ways: visit with friends, read a book, go shopping, do some volunteer work, or go to a movie. The means by which you can distract yourself are endless. *The important thing is to make a conscious effort to seek them out.*

Also important is to talk to yourself in appropriate ways. Here are some of the things you might say:

- "I don't have to reach for a pill just because I want one."
- "I can stand doing without opioid drugs, because they do not really help my pain."
- "Thinking that I need a painkiller doesn't mean I *need* one. It's only a thought. I can have the thought and let it go."

You have another weapon besides self-talk. *By working on this program, you have increased your tolerance for discomfort.* You have a greater ability to put up with annoyances and setbacks. You can think about them differently. You can understand that difficulties are normal, and that in spite of them, you *will* reach your goal of managing your pain.

Drugs That Do a Job for You
. . .

Now for the good news I promised you. Amazingly, drugs whose names have nothing to do with pain—anticonvulsants, antispasm medications, and antidepressants—can produce marvelous results for people in chronic pain.

Anticonvulsants, for example, which were originally developed to treat epilepsy, can diminish some types of "shooting" pain. Antispasm medications, also called muscle relaxers, control muscle spasm and thereby cut back on pain that stems from this source.

But the drugs that can do real wonders for chronic pain patients are, surprisingly, the antidepressants.

Why is this so?

Endorphins, the natural painkillers produced by the brain and the spinal cord, are not effective unless the brain also produces adequate levels of the natural antidepressant serotonin. People with chronic pain tend to have low levels of serotonin, just as people with depression do. (That may be one reason CPS sufferers tend to be depressed.) Antidepressant medications, by raising the amount of serotonin available to the nervous system, increase the effectiveness of endorphins and thus relieve pain.

So these drugs could just as well be called "endorphin enhancers," or the like. The point is that they are multipurpose drugs, so you don't have to be concerned about the psychological connotation of their name.

The most commonly prescribed antidepressants that are particularly good for chronic pain are Sinequan, Elavil, Pamelor, Anafranil, Norpramin, and Tofranil.

It's a good idea to talk with your physician about antidepressants and the other drugs discussed above. Not all doctors are aware of what pain specialists have discovered about the pain uses of these drugs. Most likely he or she will want to follow up on this information, but if not, you might want to review the matter with a pain medicine specialist.

My conviction is that antidepressant drugs, in particular, can be a highly valuable part of a pain management program. *One of their greatest advantages is that they can help you sleep.* Quite often, when I put patients on antidepressants, they report sleeping better almost immediately and many, within a fairly short time, are sleeping well for the first time in years.

Thomas Ivans, for example, for all of his use of painkillers and tranquilizers, and his nodding off during the day, rarely got a decent night's sleep. The first night I prescribed an antidepressant for him, he slept for seven hours straight.

That's important, because chronic pain patients need both a clear mind and a minimum of six hours of uninterrupted sleep in order to energize to fight pain. Painkillers, in addition to their other disadvantages, usually produce only fitful sleep.

So *good* sleep can be encouraged by the use of appropriate medications, but just as critical are the attitudes you develop and the actions you take in order to sleep better. We're going to talk about that now.

Getting Those Good Six Hours
• • •

Every morning I ask the patients in my program, "How did you sleep last night?" I usually hear reports of inadequate sleep, sporadic sleep, and troubled sleep. *What I hear in particular is worry over lack of sleep.* Often the worry sounds worse than the sleeplessness itself.

I remind people that a good night's sleep is important, yes, *but, ironically, you cannot get that sleep until you stop feeling tense about not getting it.* Stress, as you know, tightens your muscles and increases your pain, and pain keeps you awake.

So you have to learn to think rationally about sleep. You have to *plan* how you will handle sleep problems, rather than fussing over them.

A sleep diary, kept by your bedside for a few nights, is a good way to begin because it allows you to track what is actually going on. The diary needn't be at all formal. It can look as simple as this:

SLEEP DIARY

Date: _____

Time I got into bed: _____

Time I woke up: _____

Estimated time awake: _____

Time I woke up again: _____

Estimated time awake: _____

Time I woke up again: _____

Estimated time awake: _____

Morning wake-up time: _____

Each time you wake up, jot down the time. Of course, you'll have to wait until the next morning to estimate the amount of time you spent awake. Generally, though, people with sleeping problems glance at the clock often enough to get a fairly good idea. Add up the estimated awake times, subtract them from the number of hours between bedtime and morning wake-up time, and you'll have a handle on how much sleep you are losing. I ask you to do all this because you'll probably find, when you put it all together, that you're getting more sleep than you think.

Put the diary where you can find it easily because you'll be keeping it again after you have tried the techniques described in the next few pages. These techniques should make it possible for you to greatly increase not only the number of hours you sleep, but your hours of *uninterrupted* sleep.

As you've probably noticed, every activity in this program is directed toward consistency and function. If you want to function better, you need to work at it and to be consistent in your efforts.

These principles also apply to sleep. Even though we usually think of sleeping as doing nothing, sleeping well takes doing something. It requires putting order in your existence. If your life is disordered, your sleep will be, too.

But if you suffer from chronic pain, and particularly if you're no longer working, your life tends to become anything but orderly. Somewhere along the way you lose that sense of urgency about setting schedules and deadlines for yourself. And when you lose control over your days, you also lose control over your nights.

In a later chapter I'll tell you how to make time work for you again in performing daily activities. In the meantime, you can begin by bringing time management into your bedroom. It's fairly simple:

Rule #1: Go to bed about the same time every night.

Rule #2: Get out of bed about the same time every morning, *no matter how much sleep you have had.*

Lying in bed to "catch up" on lost sleep is a disaster because it guarantees another lost day. It also means that you will never escape the cycle of interrupted sleep.

So you have to be firm with yourself about establishing realistic hours for getting into bed and out of it. Set an alarm clock for waking up. Write your going-to-bed time on the calendar and regard it as a standing appointment. It is just as important as any other appointment you will ever make.

To encourage sleep, begin with the basics. Keep your bedroom as quiet and free of distractions as possible. If you haven't yet invested in a firm mattress, do so. (If you can see the contours of your body in the mattress, you need a firmer one.) If you suffer from neck pain, get a cervical pillow—soft in the middle with hard edges—to support your neck. For back pain, sleep on your side with a pillow between your legs or on your back with a pillow under your knees and your knees bent. These positions serve to reduce pressure on your back and to ease you into sleep.

Don't stint on making your bed attractive to you. If there are particular types of sheets and blankets you find cozy, buy them. If you have the idea you'd like a new headboard, purchase it. Anything you think may help you sleep well is worth investing in.

But don't make your bed so attractive that you want to be in it during the day.

Your bed is to be used for two things only: nighttime sleeping and sex. It is not for other activities, such as

- reading
- watching television
- working crossword puzzles
- writing letters

Nor is it for anything else that supposedly relaxes you into a good night's sleep. For one thing, reading, writing, and watching TV in bed strains your neck muscles. Moreover, these activities distract you from a major objective: *to associate bed with sleep.*

That's why it's a good idea to move a television set, reading lamp, bedside books, writing paper—except for the sleep diary and another diary I'll tell you about later—*out* of the bedroom. There's something else you have to steer clear of, too—napping.

When you sleep poorly, and you suffer from chronic pain, you may think you can make yourself feel better by "putting your feet up" every so often during the day. But napping doesn't really improve your well-being, and it actually erodes your sleep base. Most people are programmed to sleep in six- to eight-hour stretches. If you sleep in snatches during the day, it's unlikely you'll get your full complement of sleep at night.

Napping has other disadvantages, too. One nap easily leads to another, and pretty soon there can be very little left in your day *but* napping. When that happens, napping actually encourages pain by depriving you of

- social contact
- structure
- motivation
- energy

In short, napping deprives you of all the basics that you need to get better.

So if you want to succeed at managing your pain, you must work toward napping less. Cutting back on painkilling drugs can help in this regard, by the way, because you will be less tired during the day.

Don't quit napping "cold turkey." Start by limiting your naps to one a day. Psychologically, just knowing that you will be able to lie down at some point diminishes the urge to lie down. Establish a particular naptime, from three to four in the afternoon, for example, and tell yourself: That will be it. Don't watch the clock. Don't start early by taking little naps in preparation for the big nap—the way some people take small drinks to prepare for the cocktail hour. Instead, get involved in other activities. Later on, as you become less dependent on napping, it will be easier to give it up all together.

It can help to arrange your living quarters so that they are not so "nap friendly." Napping, as you know, occurs rather spontaneously when you get off your feet, so you want to limit temptation.

Keep the door to your bedroom *closed* during the day. Outside of the bedroom, put plastic covers or some other "nap aversive" covers on the sofas. Replace lounge chairs and recliners with straight-backed chairs. You can assure your family that all of this is temporary until you have broken the napping habit.

Finally, don't watch television with your feet up, or even watch too much of it with your feet on the floor, since TV, with its repetitive quality, is a great nap inducer. Be particularly wary of films you have seen many times before. After all, how many times can you watch *Sunset Boulevard* without dozing off?

Besides giving up napping, there are some simple things related to food and drink that you can do to encourage nighttime sleeping:

❑ *Eat a consistent number of meals each day.* It doesn't matter whether that's three large meals or six smaller meals, as long as you have a pattern. Consistency keeps your energy level constant and allows your body to figure out when it's time to sleep.

❏ **Consume about 70 percent of your calories at breakfast and lunch.** That way your energy level will be higher during the day and lower in the evening, making it easier to fall sleep.

❏ **Eliminate caffeine from your diet.** Caffeine can keep you from falling asleep or make you sleep erratically. And like any other stimulant, it creates highs and lows that ultimately rob you of needed energy.

❏ **Eliminate alcohol as a sleep inducer.** Alcohol has a rebound effect. It puts you to sleep for a while, then wakes you up, leaving you feeling worse. In fact, alcohol should be out of a pain-fighting diet altogether.

These suggestions can be quite helpful in reclaiming your sleep base. But you also need to know how to handle the problem that probably concerns you most: what to do when you wake up and find yourself in pain.

When Pain Is at Its Most Tyrannical
• • •

No matter how often you have been awakened this way, the experience is almost always frightening. In the dark, pain has its most potent power to terrorize. No wonder, then, that in the early morning hours catastrophizing can easily take over:

"I haven't been able to sleep a wink. I'll be absolutely wasted tomorrow."

"I'll never get a good night's sleep again."

"Lack of sleep will kill me."

When you get on a "roll" of this sort, your body tenses up, and tense muscles ensure the maintenance of poor sleep. They also ensure that the next day will be worse for you. So catastrophizing is not a helpful response to being awakened by pain.

Another response that isn't helpful is to "demand" that you fall back to sleep in spite of the pain. "I tell myself that I'm not going to tolerate being kept awake," a patient once told me. But he stayed awake nonetheless. Sleep, like relaxation, is something that you *allow* to happen, not something that you can *make* happen. And the best way to allow it to happen is to detach yourself from a preoccupation with falling asleep.

Resist the impulse to scan your body for pain. Little pains are more apparent at night, so scanning can trigger catastrophizing. Instead, go about your business, *which is to fill up the time until you naturally become sleepy again.*

If you have to urinate, go to the bathroom. If you suddenly feel wide awake, *don't go back into the bedroom.* Instead, go into another room where you can perform activities that interest you without disturbing anyone. If it's chilly in the house, take a blanket or a sweater with you.

Out of the bedroom, look for things that will distract you yet calm you down, such as reading, doing a puzzle, or watching television. This is not the time to perform your exercises, which will only invigorate you.

Don't think about *when* you are going to get tired. Concentrate on what you are doing until you *feel* yourself getting tired. This is a natural feeling, and it *will* come. When it does, get back into bed and make yourself as comfortable as you can.

Now focus on your diaphragmatic breathing, in and out, gently and deeply. Do a relaxation practice. Visualize yourself lying on warm, powdery sand, on clouds, or on some other inviting cushion that would soothe you to sleep. Pay a mental visit to that First Bank of National Resources, too, and draw out those important qualities of courage, patience, and faith. *Believing that things will improve in time can be more powerful than a sleeping pill.* These are your weapons against the midnight terrors.

If you find that you cannot fall back to sleep, leave the bedroom again and resume your activity. Even if you have to do this several times, eventually you will grow tired enough to fall asleep.

After you follow this pattern for a week or so, you will find that after you leave the bedroom you get sleepy again rather quickly. Soon you may fall back to sleep with ease without having to leave the bedroom at all.

As you go through this process, start to keep the sleep diary again. You should find that, *gradually,* the estimated amount of time you spend awake diminishes. In time you may sleep through the night.

And with the energy you gain by sleeping better and using fewer painkilling drugs, you will be more effective in taking back your life from pain.

Physiotherapy for the Mind

When we think of healing, we almost automatically think of drugs or a medical procedure. In our society we're used to handing over the curative process to somebody else or to something *outside* of ourselves, like doctors or medications.

But, as you have learned, there are other routes besides the medical. Relaxation and detachment, for example, are *inner* pathways. They begin inside you, and they grow in power as you use them. But even though you can't hold these things in your hand, the way you can hold a bottle of pills, they are just as real and often more valid when it comes to easing chronic pain.

I'm about to show you how these techniques can be expanded and used together with your imagination to utilize the curative power of your subconscious mind. The process isn't mysterious or arcane. It is simply a reality that most of us don't have much experience with. *It is inner healing by the mind.*

Why Inner Healing Works for Chronic Pain

* * *

I've said a number of times that chronic pain is a matter of perception. That means it is a very personal affair. Only your mind knows what pain—and, conversely, what comfort—means to you. So no matter how much outside assistance you may get, you must develop your own special abilities to help effect a cure.

By its very nature, the subconscious is usually hidden from us. You can access parts of it, though, by using one of your most powerful resources—imagination. Think of your imagination not as something that's simply there, but as a kind of hidden energy that you train to work for you.

When you tap into your imagination, you discover the very individual images you associate with causing pain and with stopping pain.

You can then use these and other images to create mental scenarios—stories you tell yourself in a relaxed state—that counter pain. These scenarios, though they develop out of your imagination, are not mere storytelling. On the contrary, they are a highly personalized prescription for eliminating pain.

You can't begin to eliminate something unless you know what it looks like and feels like. Right now, though, your pain is invisible to you, rather like a criminal who is unknown to the police even though several people claim to have seen him. So you have to think of yourself as one of those police artists who help out with the investigation. You have to create a composite picture of your pain, using your emotions as your brush and your imagination as your guide.

Only by doing this can you give your pain a concrete character, turn it into something that you can see with your mind's eye.

If you're not used to tapping into your imagination much, you may wonder if I'm asking you to go back to kindergarten. "What do you want from me, Doc?" a policeman once asked me. "I can't do this kind of stuff."

I told him what I'm going to tell you: Trust me. Whether you believe it or not, this works. You have to give a little, though. You have to give *up*

- judging something you haven't tried.
- holding your emotions in check.
- being stuck in one place.

Why not be open and make the choice to try this "stuff" with me? You don't have anything to lose by trying, do you?

In my program at Lenox Hill, inner healing is taught by Donald Douglas, M.D., one of the most imaginative and original thinkers in this field.

To begin with, Dr. Douglas asks our patients to draw two stick figures:

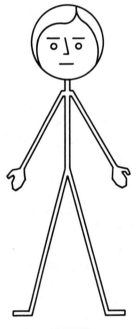

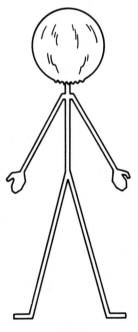

FRONT   BACK

These figures can help them make an *inner* analysis of their pain. Drawing, Dr. Douglas says, reinforces the process of looking within.

The patients circle the areas where they feel pain. Then they try to imagine the attributes of the pain tissue, not as it would exist in a physiology textbook, but as it exists in their minds.

Why don't you draw the stick figures and try to imagine the same thing? Then ask yourself, as Dr. Douglas asks our patients, "If I had to assign a color to my pain, what would it be?" Color evokes feeling and reveals emotion, so it's important to *feel* the color that's associated with the pain. If you have a crayon or Magic Marker on hand in the appropriate color, color in the pain areas you drew on the stick figures.

When Dr. Douglas does this exercise, more than half of the patients color their pain red. Red evokes danger, heightened emotion, and distress—all qualities easily associated with pain.

But even though red may be the most obvious choice, you don't have to select it for that reason. If red came into your mind —fine. If it didn't, allow yourself to find out what's really there. Let your mind follow its own path. This is *your* pain we're talking about, *your* particular curative resources we're uncovering.

After you have selected your pain's color, think about its texture. Hard or soft? Smooth or rough? How about its quality? Sharp? Dull? Nagging? Burning?

Finally, what images does your pain call to mind? "It's like a dragon breathing fire at me," one patient told Dr. Douglas. Another described his pain as "an arrow that got stuck in my back."

The first pictures that come into your head are likely to be the most powerful ones. Allow them to come forth, even if they're somewhat frightening.

What's more difficult is to imagine the healthy tissue surrounding your pain. When asked to do that, patients sometimes ask, "What healthy tissue?"

Often it's hard to remember that *most* of your body is pain free. You'll realize that, though, if you take a good look at the stick figures you drew. The pain areas you circled are probably relatively small compared to the areas you *didn't* circle.

Dr. Douglas advises patients to *think of those areas outside the circles, the healthy tissue, as having curative powers.* He emphasizes that it can be relieving to visualize the healthy tissue as moving in and replacing or transforming the pain tissue.

You can obtain relief, too, through the following steps:

First, you must let yourself believe in the power of your healthy tissue. Ask yourself:

What is its color?

What is its texture?

What qualities does it have?

After you have determined these things, think about this: If my pain were to disappear, how would that happen? How would the healthy tissue heal the pain tissue?

Here's how several patients visualized the process. The woman who imagined her pain as a fire-eating dragon—red was the way she had colored it—saw the healthy tissue as being cool blue, rather like a clear river. When she thought of healing, she saw the blue water rising and bathing the dragon so that the red fire in his mouth was gently extinguished.

The man who imagined his pain as an arrow—steel gray was the way he colored it—saw the healthy tissue as being green. When he thought of healing, he saw tall green grass growing and, with its roots, carefully lifting out the arrow and releasing it.

Dr. Douglas points out that patients' particular scenarios are up to them. Remember, though, that gentle images are the most soothing and usually the most effective as well. It's best to visualize pain as being worn away, evaporating, disintegrating, being lifted out, or something of this sort, rather than being hacked out or blown out, for example. Bear in mind, though, that a knife or a volcano may have external business to do first—if you feel the pain buried so deep within, for example, that you can only visualize it as erupting—before inner peace can prevail. Whatever you imagine must be your own in the sense that it truly fits your condition.

Putting the Scenarios to Work

• • •

Whenever you play healing images through your mind, a healing process takes place, even if you are not consciously aware of it—and even if you do not completely believe it will work.

That's because in certain ways the nervous system is really a switchboard of colors and perceptions that can be regulated by your visualization so that a calm, healing energy moves through the body.

You can influence your nervous system in the interests of feeling better. But you must take the time to work the switchboard. So it's important to sit down in a quiet place a few times each day, with your eyes closed, and run the healing images through your mind, as if you were in a movie theater of your own construction. See the healthy tissue at work as it takes over the pain tissue and replaces it, in whatever way you have imagined. By imagining, you can *make* this happen, not immediately and perhaps not completely, but in time you will notice significant improvement.

Like the "relaxation moments," these "movie breaks" needn't take long. But since their effect is cumulative, the more daily breaks you can take, the calmer and more at ease you will feel.

As you begin to appreciate the value of these breaks, you will realize that you can go even further in unleashing the inner forces of your mind to achieve what Dr. Douglas calls "a permanent state of comfort." Imaging, he says, is like a soothing blanket that you weave around yourself and for yourself. And you can make the "comfort" blanket larger and more effective.

Comfort, like motivation, is something that chronic pain patients must have. It's the staging platform from which healing takes place.

But when you suffer from chronic pain, it's difficult to feel comfortable. Unless you can achieve comfort, though, your energy level will remain low, no matter how motivated you are to fight pain. *You need significantly more comfort than motivation to energize yourself.* To express that idea, Dr. Douglas utilizes (with apologies to Albert Einstein) the following equation:

$$\text{ENERGY} = \text{MOTIVATION} \times \text{COMFORT}^2$$

Fortunately, as you have already seen from relaxation and imaging, you have the power to move yourself into a more comfortable state.

But there's a way to combine both of these techniques so that you can achieve yet another level of comfort. This blending can carry you to a place deep inside yourself where comfort is generated —and suggestions for future healing abound. That place is really a land of treasures, and when you travel there, you are invited to scoop them up and take them home to make your life better.

If you believe that such a place exists—and every good feeling you've ever had in your entire life tells you that it does—I'm asking you to embark on a journey, *on a road that replaces pain with peace.*

The Comfort Road
. . .

Benita Galway, who had been an administrator in the same accounting firm for twenty-five years, was reluctant to go on any trips to a place she wasn't sure existed. "It all sounds like nonsense to me," she said, resting her head against the back of her chair to alleviate her neck pain. Benita was wound up tighter than a drum, yet she resisted any of the so-called mental techniques in the program, arguing that there was nothing wrong with her mind. I assured her that I quite agreed, I simply wanted her to recognize the *powers* of her mind.

"But how can I think about being somewhere else when I'm hurting so much?" Benita asked me.

"It's *because* you are hurting so much that I want you to try being somewhere else," I replied.

"Well," Benita said, thinking it over, "I just can't see how it's possible."

The answer, I told Benita, lay in that unique ability of human beings to detach mentally from one place and be in another at the same time. For example, you are reading this book right now, but you may also be listening to a conversation in the next room or keeping one eye on the television set.

We constantly make "mental trips" from one focus to another and from one reality to another, from the past to the present, for example, or the present to the future.

At the same time, we have the capacity to detach from many of the sensory stimuli around us, simply because there are so many of them. For example, you probably aren't noticing the pressure of your thumb on this book or the heaviness of your shoes.

So we can block out some things, and we can also focus on more than one thing. One ability reinforces the other. And when we take advantage of both, we find that we can reach yet another reality—the healing one that is inside of us.

Just like everything else in this program, inner healing is achieved in stages. Dr. Douglas describes the stages this way:

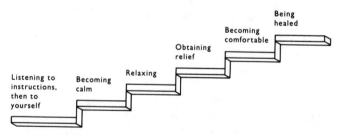

You listen to what you tell yourself in order to become calm and relaxed—detaching from sensation. Then you create and visualize the images you need to become comfortable and healed, putting yourself in another place while still being where you are. The steps involved will become apparent if you do the following inner healing practice, as developed by Dr. Douglas at Lenox Hill Hospital.

The first time you perform the practice, it's best to have someone else read it to you in a quiet, calm voice, so that you can concentrate on following the instructions and then on "seeing" the pictures that are created. If no one is available to help you, read through the entire practice a few times until you understand the way it works.

Pay attention to remembering the details of the scenario. Many of the images in it are symbols of pain and of healing. Later on I'll explain what the symbols mean. And I'll tell you how, based on Dr. Douglas's principles, you can use them to create scenarios of your own. In the meantime, though, concentrate on working with this model practice.

Breathing Out the Past, Breathing In the Present
. . .

Sit on a comfortable chair with your hands on your lap, palms facing up. (If you're more comfortable standing or lying down, that's all right, too.) Let your body be as loose as possible. The room should be reasonably quiet, but it doesn't have to be noise free. Don't attempt to block out any noises. Simply let them be.

Close your eyes and keep them closed for the entire practice.
You are ready to begin.
Breathe in and out deeply a few times.
Tighten the muscles of your big toes—count one . . . two . . . three . . . four . . . five—and let go.
Tighten the muscles of your calves—count one . . . two . . . three . . . four . . . five—and let go.
Tighten the muscles of your thighs (by pressing your feet down on the floor)—count one . . . two . . . three . . . four . . . five —and let go.
Tighten your abdominal muscles—count one . . . two . . . three . . . four . . . five—and let go.

Continue by tightening and then releasing the muscles of your neck, face, shoulders, and forearms, each to a slow count of five.

Remember to breathe deeply, in and out.

You are breathing *out* the past and breathing *in* the present. You are letting go of clocks and calendars. You are letting go.

You feel a tingling sensation in your fingers, elbows, forearms, and shoulders. Embrace that feeling. Let it travel anywhere in your body.

You notice that your palms have become warm.

Allow all of the tension in your body to flow into your palms so that your fists close. When your muscles are ready, you'll find that your fingers can open with no effort on your part.

Now focus on visualizing the letters of the alphabet, one at a time, from A to Z.

See each letter in large type, small type, or both—Aa, Bb, Cc, and so forth—the way the letters looked when you first learned to write in school. See yourself writing on the blackboard.

As the letters float past you, continue to breathe deeply. You are breathing out the tensions of the past and present. You are breathing in the calm that is waiting for you in the future.

Visualize the number 1. You are on the landing of a stairway or in an elevator on the ground floor. As you ascend, slowly count the numbers—1, 2, 3, 4—all the way to 10.

When you reach the top, start to descend slowly, in an elevator or on the stairs, counting backward and seeing the numbers—10, 9, 8, 7—and so forth, all the way down to 1.

When you get to the ground floor, you notice that there is a door in front of you. You go through the door, and you enter a beautiful place.

It is a garden on a bright, sunny day, lush with green grass and bright flowers. You notice a thick grove of evergreens on your right, with birds flying through the branches.

Your senses go back to a summer's day like this one. You see the colors of the garden; you feel the soft texture of the grass; you smell the flowers. You absorb the healing energy of the place. You can sense good cells replacing the bad ones in your body.

Now you notice that there is a wide prairie behind the garden. A long time ago a meteor struck one section of the prairie and created a deep, barren pit. But in time, bit by bit, fresh pieces of earth, carried by the wind, filled up the pit and made it just like the rest of the prairie surrounding it. Now the entire area is fertile and growing as it used to be. You can hardly see where the pit was.

In time, also, melting ice and rain created a gentle river that runs through the prairie. This river is also irrigating the garden. The river is a stream of comfort. You can feel its comfort wind around your body, soft as cotton, strong as steel, to protect you.

The people who live on the prairie send a guide to meet you. The guide leads you over a row of stepping-stones into a deep forest. He takes you up a green hill to a sparkling waterfall, where jewels of wisdom are yours for the taking. Behind the waterfall you meet a child, the spiritual aspects of yourself when you were younger. "Can you help me?" you ask the child. The child says, "Yes." You reply, "I am your older self, and I can help you, too. You need not suffer anymore."

At the edge of the forest you see a time train waiting. You board the train with the child, knowing that you can go back and forth—from past to present to future—at will. In the past, the child helps you gather up the good feelings you can remember from loving relationships and happy events. You experience these emotions now. And you realize that you can take them with you to the future, where things will be better for you.

As you think of this, you are back in the garden again. You feel its healing energy moving through your body. You realize that nothing else and no one else can bring on this healing state better than you can. *Nothing else and no one else.*

Slowly open your eyes. Close them again for a moment. Take a deep breath. Prepare to keep the relaxation and comfort within your body. Then allow yourself, gradually, to become aware of the things around you. You have returned from the inner journey.

The inner journey, as I noted earlier, is physiotherapy for the nervous system, an exercise for the mind. As with the exercises and the relaxation technique you learned earlier, the inner journey requires daily practice. The more you practice, the more easily you can take part in the journey, and the more you can do with it. You will become adept, for example, at creating scenarios of your own and at planting pain-fighting images in your mind.

These images are suggestions. Once planted, they can go to work whenever you need them during the day, without conscious effort on your part. They can enable you to perform activities with far greater ease and in a more pain-free manner. For example, if while on the journey you see yourself raking up leaves in a pleasant setting with feelings of buoyancy and well-being, these feelings will be there when you have to perform the actual task.

But to gain the full value of the journey, if you choose to do it, the process has to become almost second nature. That means you must practice for fifteen minutes to half an hour every day. Two journeys in a row are the most effective.

Any time is a good time to practice. In the morning the journey can energize you. Before going to bed it can relax you and also chart the course for the next day's activities. It can also be helpful to do a journey when you wake up at night and have difficulty falling back to sleep.

The more imaginative you are, the more easily you will catch on to this, so try to release that inner child who used to enjoy "making believe."

If you are particularly gifted at imagining, you may be that one person in ten who is able to say "My pain stopped" after the first practice. One man who was severely crippled saw himself as a cloud rising above his pain. An artist visualized the colors on her palette as mechanisms for dissolving her pain. Both of these patients became pain free almost immediately.

But most people, says Dr. Douglas, need at least four or five sessions before they begin to notice greater comfort and healing. Benita Galway, to her amazement, felt an improvement after only two sessions, and now she is an enthusiastic practitioner of these journeys.

So let me repeat these now familiar words of advice:

- You need to be open.
- You need to be patient.
- You need to work slowly.
- You need to put up with setbacks.

Finally, you need to be aware that, as when you are doing the relaxation technique, unexpected feelings may emerge. We'll talk about what they mean in a later chapter. For now, just remember that they are nothing to fear. Allow them to happen, if they do—and continue on your journey.

Types of Imagery
. . .

The scenarios you devise will arise naturally out of your imagination. But you are looking for guided imagery—imagery that fights pain—so Dr. Douglas advises that you try to include certain elements:

❏ *A comforting environment.* Focus on images that promote well-being, such as the lush garden in the practice above. A garden, with its summer beauty—trees, flowers, and birds—evokes the sensory responses and positive feelings that heal. Being in full bloom, it also conveys the idea that life constantly renews itself, as you will be renewed when you triumph over pain.

❏ *Symbols of healing.* Create images that symbolize your pain and the healthy tissue that will heal it. In the practice, for example, the meteor pit stands for pain, and the fresh earth that fills it in represents healing tissue. Examples of healing images include a soft rain dissolving the thorns on a rose or waves lapping gently at burning sand and making it disappear.

❏ *The idea of gradualism.* In the practice, the meteor pit gets filled in *bit by bit.* This image plants the suggestion that chronic pain gets better in steps—in time. This is important because chronic pain engenders impatience, which triggers muscular ten-sion and increased pain. So you have to remind yourself by all means possible—and images are good ones—that slow and steady does it.

❑ *Time travel.* You may not have had much to feel good about lately, but in the past you probably did. If you can retrieve those positive feelings, you can use them to comfort yourself now. In the practice, the image of the time train allows you to do that. But a car, plane, magic carpet, or some other form of transportation would work just as well. If you wish, your spiritual child, the most feeling part of you, can accompany you when journeying in time.

Don't forget to travel to the future, too, says Dr. Douglas, because that is the place of recovery. In the practice, the future is conveyed by walking along *a row of stepping-stones* into the forest and *up a green hill* to the waterfall. Such images remind you that with diligence and hard work, you will come to a better place.

❑ *Your own power.* The practice ends with the statement that *nothing else and no one else can create this healing state, only you.* There are many ways to phrase this take-charge concept or to visualize it—you in the role of president, for example, or as leader of an orchestra—but no matter how you envision it, try to work this idea into each healing journey. It's a very powerful idea because it is true.

There are several other things you can do to enhance the effec-tiveness of your imaging, Dr. Douglas points out. One is to use puns or double meanings. For example, as you visualize the number *1* (one), you can tell yourself, What I have *won.* As you visualize the letter *B,* you can think, What can *be* (the future). The letter C can be *see,* as in seeing inside yourself. As you gain experience in journeying, such associations will just "pop" into your mind, as will the scenarios themselves.

Another imaging device—and you can use this one during a journey or at any time—is to make use of bodily metaphors. Let's say, for example, that you suddenly feel "a knot" developing in your stomach. Instead of becoming panicky, you visualize the knot tying up the pain in your back and carrying the pain away. Or if you've done something forgetful and think you have a "hole" in your head, you can visualize the hole expanding and swallowing up the pain you feel in your shoulders.

As you can see, imaging has endless possibilities. But the most compelling thing about it is that it is your *personal* message to pain —it fits the contours of your mind just the way a tailor-made suit or dress fits your body.

So it's worthwhile suspending whatever disbelief you may have until you've really given it a try—and by a try, I mean daily practices for at least two weeks or so.

The inner journeys are like planting seeds. Those seeds need time to gestate, but the gestation period—hidden from us—is just as significant as the period of visible growth. As with seeds, you have to have faith that something is growing before you actually see it.

A concluding thought: Even though the inner journey takes place in your head, that doesn't mean the pain is "all in your head." I bring this point up again because you don't need to give yourself an additional guilt trip. The truth is that imaging and the inner journey, like the other techniques in this program, work only on *real* pain. Your pain is real, and it *can* be managed.

Now we are going to talk about how you can make a pain-fighting device out of something that may be fighting you right now: the clock.

Putting Time on Your Side

Time can be your enemy—or it can be the enemy of your pain. It's as simple as that. And learning to turn time against pain is what this chapter is all about.

Unless you control time in a way that fights your pain, time works against you. That's a depressing thought, because you can't get better without having time as an ally. So if you suspect that you and time are on the outs, you need to begin the reconciliation process now. You need to learn time management.

Time management? you may ask. Isn't that something that's used in business to increase productivity? What does time management have to do with chronic pain?

The answer is: Everything. Because managing time *is* managing pain to a very large extent.

And that holds true whether you are working or whether you have lots of time on your hands. *In fact, the more free time you have, the more important time management becomes.* Without structure, your life can get caught in a warp. Time itself flattens out and becomes shapeless, like a drooping clock in a Salvador Dalí painting. Your job now, if you choose to learn time management, is to make that clock round and dimensional again. When you do that, you revive time. You breathe life into it, so that it can breathe life into you.

Getting Out of the Warp

· · ·

What do you do all day?

Though most CPS sufferers think they have an answer to that question, the truth is they have only a general idea, such as "I go to the office, I spend time with my family, I watch TV, and I go to sleep" or "I try to keep busy, I do a little shopping, I prepare dinner, I read for a while, and I go to sleep."

Contrast these two statements with the following statement from Chuck Bowers, an unmarried dental technician in my program: "I get up at six-thirty, do my exercises, and go for a walk. Before I have breakfast at eight, I take a shower. By nine, I'm in the laboratory working on dental molds. Lunchtime, I usually run errands, and if I have time, I visit an invalid aunt who lives in the neighborhood. After work, three days a week, I spend an hour as a volunteer in the literacy program at the local library. I get home around seven, eat a TV dinner, and usually spend an hour or two at a neighborhood social club until I go to sleep."

The first two statements are vague. Chuck Bowers, on the other hand, knows exactly what he does and for how long. So, if questioned on the subject, Chuck can be precise about when pain prevented him from carrying out an activity, such as visiting his aunt, or when pain developed in the course of an activity, such as working in his lab. Chuck has the basic data he needs to put time and pain together.

By creating a time/activity/pain chart (we'll call it TAP) you can track, over the course of a week, all the major activities you perform. You can also measure, by means of visual analog scales, what effect these activities have on your pain.

For each *waking* hour of the day, note your activities, the pain level you felt at the start of each activity (PLS), and the pain level you felt at completion (PLC).

A daily entry can look like this:

(Time/Activity/Pain) TAP CHART

DATE: _____

		(Pain Level Start)	(Pain Level Completion)

7 A.M.   Activities

——————————— PLS ├────┤ PLC ├──────┤

——————————— PLS ├────┤ PLC ├──────┤

——————————— PLS ├────┤ PLC ├──────┤

8 A.M.   Activities

——————————— PLS ├────┤ PLC ├──────┤

——————————— PLS ├────┤ PLC ├──────┤

——————————— PLS ├────┤ PLC ├──────┤

9 A.M.   Activities

——————————— PLS ├────┤ PLC ├──────┤

——————————— PLS ├────┤ PLC ├──────┤

——————————— PLS ├────┤ PLC ├──────┤

10 A.M.   Activities

——————————— PLS ├────┤ PLC ├──────┤

——————————— PLS ├────┤ PLC ├──────┤

——————————— PLS ├────┤ PLC ├──────┤

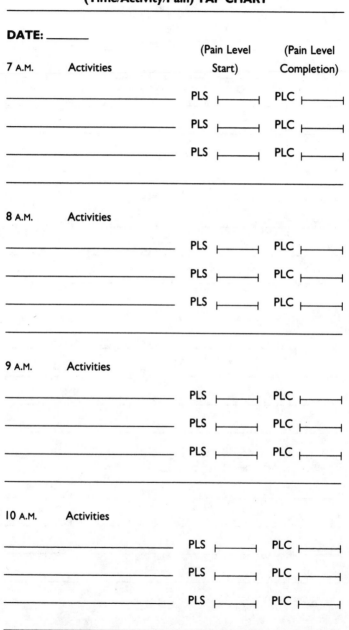

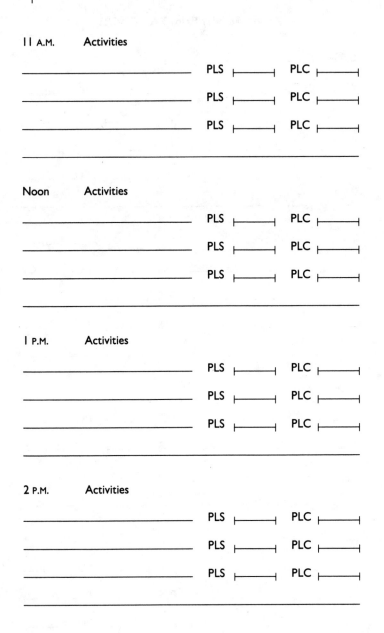

11 A.M.　　**Activities**

_____ PLS ├──────┤ PLC ├──────┤

_____ PLS ├──────┤ PLC ├──────┤

_____ PLS ├──────┤ PLC ├──────┤

Noon　　**Activities**

_____ PLS ├──────┤ PLC ├──────┤

_____ PLS ├──────┤ PLC ├──────┤

_____ PLS ├──────┤ PLC ├──────┤

1 P.M.　　**Activities**

_____ PLS ├──────┤ PLC ├──────┤

_____ PLS ├──────┤ PLC ├──────┤

_____ PLS ├──────┤ PLC ├──────┤

2 P.M.　　**Activities**

_____ PLS ├──────┤ PLC ├──────┤

_____ PLS ├──────┤ PLC ├──────┤

_____ PLS ├──────┤ PLC ├──────┤

3 P.M.   Activities

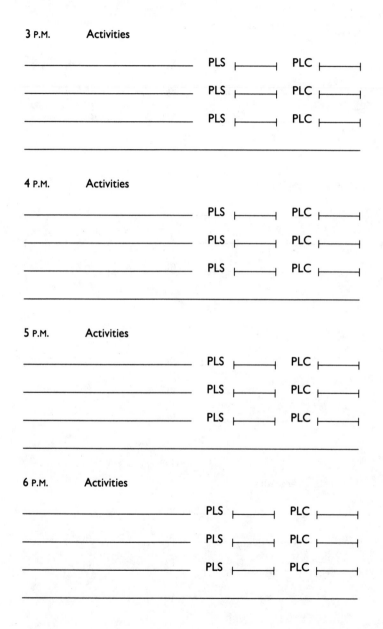

_____ PLS ⊢———⊣ PLC ⊢———⊣

_____ PLS ⊢———⊣ PLC ⊢———⊣

_____ PLS ⊢———⊣ PLC ⊢———⊣

4 P.M.   Activities

_____ PLS ⊢———⊣ PLC ⊢———⊣

_____ PLS ⊢———⊣ PLC ⊢———⊣

_____ PLS ⊢———⊣ PLC ⊢———⊣

5 P.M.   Activities

_____ PLS ⊢———⊣ PLC ⊢———⊣

_____ PLS ⊢———⊣ PLC ⊢———⊣

_____ PLS ⊢———⊣ PLC ⊢———⊣

6 P.M.   Activities

_____ PLS ⊢———⊣ PLC ⊢———⊣

_____ PLS ⊢———⊣ PLC ⊢———⊣

_____ PLS ⊢———⊣ PLC ⊢———⊣

7 P.M.   Activities

———————————————————   PLS ├——————┤   PLC ├——————┤

———————————————————   PLS ├——————┤   PLC ├——————┤

———————————————————   PLS ├——————┤   PLC ├——————┤

_____

8 P.M.   Activities

———————————————————   PLS ├——————┤   PLC ├——————┤

———————————————————   PLS ├——————┤   PLC ├——————┤

———————————————————   PLS ├——————┤   PLC ├——————┤

_____

9 P.M.   Activities

———————————————————   PLS ├——————┤   PLC ├——————┤

———————————————————   PLS ├——————┤   PLC ├——————┤

———————————————————   PLS ├——————┤   PLC ├——————┤

_____

10 P.M.   Activities

———————————————————   PLS ├——————┤   PLC ├——————┤

———————————————————   PLS ├——————┤   PLC ├——————┤

———————————————————   PLS ├——————┤   PLC ├——————┤

_____

Keep up the diary for a full week, even though you may feel some resistance to it. There's a natural tendency to balk at record keeping. But, remember, nothing recorded, nothing learned.

What you want to learn is your activity pattern—*how* you do things—and, also, *what* you are doing. Let's talk about the *how* first and then go on to the *what*.

Your activity pattern can reveal whether or not you are fighting pain effectively. Most likely you are not, since very few CPS sufferers establish the proper patterns. The majority fall into one of three "losing" patterns. Do you recognize yourself in any of them?

❑ *"As long as I keep moving, I'm okay."* You try to stay ahead of your pain by doing more and more. You think that's the way to ward pain off and, ultimately, to get better. Since you don't stop *before* pain sets in, your visual analog scales invariably show a substantial increase in pain at the completion of a task. Your week looks like this:

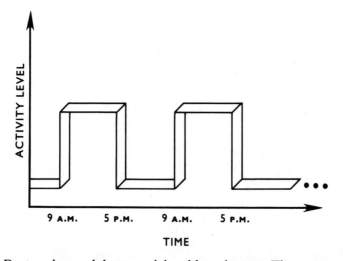

During the workday, you labor like a beaver. Then you come home and collapse into bed. But even though you *seem* to be functioning, you'll never really get better working at this pace. You need to *temper* your activity in a sensible way, which I will explain later.

❏ *"If I don't do anything, I won't hurt."* You engage in infrequent and halfhearted spurts of activity, then lapse into lethargy when the visual analog scales confirm an increase in pain. Your day is chock full of pain behaviors and pain thoughts. "Poor me" could be your middle name. Your week looks like this:

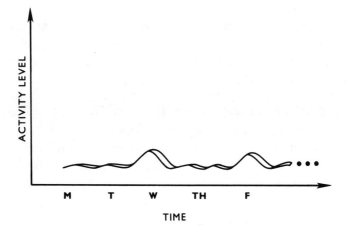

That almost horizontal line is your giveaway. *Nobody gets better by giving up.* You need to *increase* your activity level in a sensible way, which I will explain later.

❏ *"When I don't have any pain, I can make up for lost time."*
With you, it's all or nothing. One day you feel pretty good, so you
work overtime at your job, clean the apartment, and bathe the
dogs. Your visual analog scales may not show much of a pain increase that day, but the next day is another story. You catastrophize
in a major way: "I've killed myself." "I'll never be able to do
anything again." So you do almost nothing for the next few days.
Then it's up, up, and away again. Your week looks like this:

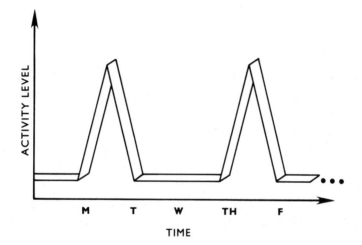

You are exhibiting the yo-yo syndrome. This pattern of activity
is so common among patients that one might even say it is an
underpinning of chronic pain. So before we talk about what you
could be doing, let's look at the life of a yo-yo. Perhaps it will sound
familiar.

Up and Down on a String

· · ·

For Rita Dawson, the yo-yo syndrome predated her chronic pain. Even in college, Rita, an elementary school teacher, had been the kind of student who stays up all night writing a paper and then collapses in bed the next day. When Rita developed back pain, she thought she could use her "catch up" abilities to help her cope. She'd spend all day Saturday sitting at her desk grading papers, for example, then lie on the sofa for most of Sunday.

If she felt better, she'd rush around Sunday night trying to "get a jump" on housework in order to be ready for—you guessed it—a thoroughly painful Monday. As Rita's pain increased, her ability to function in the classroom suffered, and she began to worry about having to leave her job.

When she joined my program, Rita was still hopping up and down on a string, unable to see that as a major source of her problems. She was feeling so bad, though, that she was willing to listen to me.

I explained to Rita that being a yo-yo began with her pattern of thinking. Her thoughts probably went something like this:

- I *should* be able to do my work the way I used to before I had pain.
- I *can't stand* not taking the opportunity to get everything done when I feel less pain.
- If I feel well, I can't relax on a weekend because I always *have* to catch up.

You probably recognize, from our earlier discussion about beliefs that make pain worse, that Rita was caught in a few booby traps. She was indulging in "should" thinking and impatient "I can't stand" thinking—both distortions that have little to do with reality. And it was these distortions that kept the yo-yo bouncing.

What Rita needed to do was to put these thoughts aside and develop new ones, based on the reality of how we disassociate activity from pain. That reality is called "gradation."

Gradation: The Only Sure Way to Be Pain Free
• • •

Rita Dawson feared that she might never be able to mark papers again, because she couldn't sit at a desk for too long. Chuck Bowers thought he might have to stop playing pool at the neighborhood social club, because he couldn't stay on his feet for too long. Deirdre Howard, a sales representative, worried that she might have to stop taking walks with her two daughters, because walking for too long a time caused pain.

Yet today Rita, Chuck, and Deirdre are all performing the activities they thought they would not be able to do. *And they no longer feel pain while doing them.*

It seems amazing. Yet it's really quite simple.

Rita, Chuck, and Deirdre learned how to break the association between pain and the activity. They learned how to practice gradation.

Gradation consists of increasing your level of activity in increments and staying at each new level for some time before climbing to the next one. It's a series of steps, with plateaus in between, rather like climbing a staircase very slowly—and pausing for a time on each stair—so that you do not get out of breath.

A graded pattern of activity looks like this:

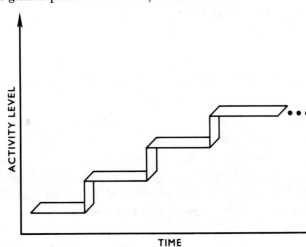

Look at the diagram and you can see that the secret of gradation lies in its slowness and sureness. When you are slow and sure, pain does not have a chance to intervene. And, eventually, your mind gives up the idea that pain has to occur. *In short, you head off trouble before it has a chance to start.*

Here is how gradation works:

1. You figure out how long you can do an activity—walking, for example—before experiencing pain or an increase in pain. This becomes your baseline for that particular activity.

2. You begin the gradation pattern by doing the activity at half of baseline.

3. In *very* small increments, you increase the amount of time, until you reach baseline.

4. In *very* small increments, you work on expanding the baseline.

In other words, you take small—but powerful—baby steps. You *adapt* to the way you must function to defeat pain.

This is how Rita Dawson learned to mark papers without pain.

I asked Rita to keep track of how long she could sit at her desk before she noticed back pain setting in. The average time—the baseline—turned out to be twenty minutes.

I told Rita to begin by marking papers for only ten minutes at a time. After that, since sitting is the least comfortable position for most people with back pain, she had to take a break and walk around. Then she could go back to the paper marking for another ten minutes. The goal, I said, was *to disassociate activity from pain by stopping the activity well before the pain set in.*

A week later Rita moved on to marking papers for twelve-minute periods, a week later to fourteen-minute periods, and so forth, until she reached the baseline. After a few weeks at baseline, she was able to go further but would always take a brief break for relaxing and limbering after thirty minutes.

A graded pattern of the sort that Rita developed should be applied to all of your major activities. Even with a hectic business schedule, you must find a way to *pace* yourself by working within a comfortable parameter.

Think of every task you do as having a red light attached to it. You want to stop before that light flashes or even before a yellow warning light goes on. So pay attention to the way you feel when you do something and pay particular attention to the heightened stress level that often precedes pain. Acknowledge it. Listen to your body, and you'll be able to catch on to gradation.

Those Two "P" Words

• • •

Gradation is just one major element of time/pain management. The other two are *planning* and *prioritizing.* Let's talk about planning first, because it is basic to everything else.

"All I can plan to do is pray that I survive," Deirdre Howard, a sales representative, told me.

Deirdre had a highly stressful, competitive job, and in addition to that, she was a single mother. She juggled a crowded monthly schedule of business trips and a household that often had to be run long distance. On top of all this, she had to cope with chronic pain, which she feared might torpedo her unsteady ship at any moment. Small wonder that Deirdre's idea of planning was just to hang on.

"There's no way you can convince me that I have time for this stuff," Deirdre insisted. "I'm totally out of control."

I told Deirdre that planning—and nothing but planning—would put her *in control* for the first time in years. In fact, the planning process in and of itself could make her feel *physically* better, just because she would be taking charge.

Deirdre's schedule, like that of many busy people with CPS, was totally out of balance.

I knew that if she understood the importance of balance, she could change her life and greatly relieve her pain. *Balance is the philosophical counterpart of gradation.* It keeps you from going too far, too fast—from doing too much, too often. And, as we discussed earlier, it actually serves to detach you from pain.

Balance can be achieved by asking yourself these three questions: What do I *have* to do? What do I *want* to do? What can I do to *relax*?

When these three elements get *equal* attention from you, you have made a powerful pain-fighting tool out of time.

So with the concept of balance in mind, examine your TAP charts. Look hard at the types of things you are doing. Recognize any lack of balance.

Then, on a piece of paper, write down your have-tos, want-tos, and relaxers for tomorrow. And make it a habit to create a schedule for each day thereafter.

It was a struggle for Deirdre, as it is for many people, to obtain balance. Her little black appointment book was full of have-tos without any want-tos or relaxers. "That's not good enough," I told her.

We set to work figuring out which have-tos could be delegated to others (even to Deirdre's daughters, Krista and Ann, who were old enough to perform some household chores). We uncovered a few have-tos that could be demoted to "have to sometime or other." And by clearing the decks a bit, we made room for the want-tos.

Want-tos were something Deirdre hadn't thought about for some time. The minute she let them cross her mind, she felt excited; she felt happy; *she felt less pain.* The same held true of relaxers, even though it was difficult for Deirdre to convince herself that they really were important. But she did, and she came up with the following schedule for the first workday after she completed my program:

Things I Have to Do	**Things I Want to Do**	**Relaxers**
Complete presentation for board meeting in Chicago.	Investigate course on interactive TV sales.	Watch TV with Krista and Ann.
Develop sales figures for departmental report.	Take Tom to lunch for his birthday.	Soak in hot tub at the spa.
Go over graphics for L.A. meeting.	Help Krista rehearse part for school play.	Begin to read new Stephen King best-seller.
Make ten cold sales calls.	Meet with interior decorator re kitchen redesign.	Chat on phone with Sally.

Your day may be very different from Deirdre's. You may work in another field. You may not be working at all. It doesn't matter. *If you're alive, you need to plan.* And then you need to look at your plan and decide which things to do first.

Deciding What to Do First

• • •

Prioritizing is based on the principle that you probably can't do everything you planned, so you have to put your energy where it counts most. *And, since chronic pain has already severely limited your energy, prioritizing has to be a priority with you.*

You must prioritize within each category, even if it means letting go of some have-tos. Better, for example, to leave a project incomplete than to miss out on a rare chance to go to the movies with friends. *You need the balance more than you need to do a perfect job.*

As you establish priorities, be aware that the parts of this program that you have decided to do belong in the "have to" category. Exercises, body awareness, relaxation practices, the inner journey of the mind—these things need to be on your schedule.

A patient will sometimes tell me that there "isn't time for all of this" (even though the actual expenditure of time, when you think about it, is rather minimal). When I hear that, I know that the person has failed to recognize his top priority. *Nothing is more important right now than getting better.* Whatever has to be done to get your life up and running again—has to be done.

Fortunately, the work of an Italian economist of the late nineteenth century can make prioritizing easier for you.

Vilfredo Pareto discovered that in any given group of items, only a small portion are significant. Pareto's principle—also called the 80/20 rule—says that, most often, *doing 20 percent of the activities on your schedule will produce 80 percent of the desired result.*

For people with chronic pain, this is very good news—so good, in fact, that I call it the "Pain-reto principle."

When used properly, Pain-reto can free you from guilt, tension, exhaustion—and other miserable pain-activating triggers. It is particularly valuable for people who try to do too much, such as the "yo-yos."

For example, straightening up a few key rooms, spraying a room freshener, and buying some flowers can accomplish 80 percent of making a house look presentable for guests. Soliciting the most likely 20 percent of potential clients can bring in 80 percent of the new clients you need. Researching the most pertinent 20 percent of sources can account for 80 percent of the success of the report.

The way to use Pain-reto, advises Jane Prawda, a dedicated occupational therapist on my staff, is to look for that vital 20 percent of your scheduled activities that will do the most good. If necessary, limit yourself to them.

That's not always easy, Jane tells patients. A congenital over-doer like Rita Dawson, for example, found it hard to do less and still feel good about herself. But she learned to accept the fact that she was not the same person she was before chronic pain. She learned to find satisfaction in being the best that she could be right now and in using every tool at her disposal—including prioritizing—to help accomplish that.

Before we part from Pain-reto, I should say that this principle should not be applied with too much zest by those who exhibit the "if I don't do anything, I won't hurt" pattern of activity. Twenty percent of nothing is still nothing. The "don't do" people need to increase activity by taking a good look at what is holding them back. One of the problems they are likely to find is that age-old time killer: procrastination.

Pain and Procrastination: An Unholy Combination
• • •

Procrastination means that you plan to do something—you schedule it, you think about it—but somehow it never gets done. You wait until later, wait until you're ready, wait until your pain stops, and so on.

Gradation is taking small steps. Procrastination, on the other hand, is taking no steps at all, and it puts the brakes on getting better.

By keeping you inactive, procrastination serves as a seedbed for pain. You have nothing to do but catastrophize. The clock sags.

All this would be bad enough, but procrastination has another twist: it makes you feel guilty all the time. Your muscles tense, and your stress level rises. In short, even though you may be lying on a sofa doing nothing, *procrastination is a major pain-activating trigger.*

You have to do something about it, even if you feel totally stuck.

Procrastination begins, as many problems do, with your thoughts, which means it's here that you must concentrate first. I don't know why, but procrastination seems to be fueled by many distortions. Maybe it takes a lot of unreal thinking to stop action, which is, after all, a normal human tendency.

You need to identify the pain-promoting thoughts that have locked you in place, recognize them as distortions (it can help to refer to our discussion of failed coping mechanisms in step 5), and replace them with pain-overcoming thoughts.

One thing that's easy to procrastinate about is doing exercises. So, as an example, let's see what kinds of thoughts can get in the way of that activity and how you can alter them:

Pain-Promoting Thoughts	Underlying Distortions	Pain-Overcoming Thoughts
I can put off exercising until later, when I'll feel like it.	I have to feel like doing something before I can act.	It's not necessary to feel like acting to make a start. Motivation will come later.
With this pain, I can't do the exercises the way I should be able to.	There is only one acceptable way to do things.	I don't have to do everything perfectly. I'll just do the best I can.
Exercising is silly. If I'm going to get better, I'll get better without it.	I'll keep doing things my way, even though it hasn't helped me so far.	I would prefer to be able to get better without exercise, but I can't. Getting better takes effort. Starting now is in my interest.

I've loused up everything else, I'll probably louse this up, too.

I'm in pain and I'm defective, and it's my own fault. I'll never be able to make my life better.

I could have done some things better, but so could everyone else. I have to start where I am now.

Exercises take too long to have an effect.

If I don't see results right away, it's not worth doing.

Pain gets better in small steps, so I have to be patient. I have to appreciate small successes.

Every time you find yourself procrastinating, dig for the thoughts that are holding you back. *Force those thoughts into the daylight and make them stand up for themselves. Most likely they can't —and you'll be prepared to replace them.*

As you can see, all of the thoughts in the right-hand column are oriented toward problem solving. They encourage you to make a start. There are several other techniques, too, that can help to overcome procrastination, as Jane Prawda points out to our patients.

One is the so-called Swiss cheese method, developed by time management expert, Alan Lakein. This consists of making small holes in a task—breaking it down into manageable parts and then working on only one part at a time.

Also effective is the "act as if" approach, which we have used several times in this book. "Act as if" you want to do something, make a start, and you will find that action is a great motivator.

Another good motivator, if you've been putting off a task, is to visualize yourself doing it in one of your "movie breaks" or while on an inner journey of the mind. These visualizations can pay off in greater focus and freedom from distorting thoughts. After visualizing, you can find that a task that was previously difficult to contemplate has become rather easy to get under way.

It can also help to promise yourself a small reward, something you'll really enjoy getting or doing, whenever you complete a task you didn't want to begin. By the way, napping and watching television don't count!

Gradation, planning for balance, prioritizing, and overcoming procrastination are also rewards in themselves, because they get the clock working for you again. Every minute is another opportunity to get better, *if* you take advantage of it.

And every task you have to do or want to do is also a chance to get better, *if* you perform it in a way that decreases pain. By combining body awareness with a practical knowledge of lifting, pushing, pulling, and so forth, you can do just that. In the next chapter I'll give you what's probably the most important physics lesson you ever had.

The Physics of Movement

Lou Kostovich, a stock analyst, loved to spend weekends puttering around his boat. One Sunday morning, as Lou picked up a pile of boards to repair the deck, he heard a "pop" and felt a searing pain in his back. A few months later the pain still hadn't gone away.

Lou had an explanation. "I just bent over, Doctor," he told me, "and a disk went out."

I hear explanations like that one all the time.

"I just reached up to get some files, and I pulled something."

"I picked up the laundry basket, and something just locked."

"I was carrying a pile of newspapers, and somehow my neck got twisted."

As you probably know by now, weak muscles are one of the causes behind these "pulls," "locks," and "twists."

But another major cause is the way these tasks were performed.

Chances are that Lou Kostovich bent over to pick up the boards without bending his knees, so that his back had to do most of the work. The physiological fact is that the back wasn't meant for lifting. Yet we use our backs to lift things all the time. Not only do we lift things improperly, we often do these things wrong, too:

- Standing
- Sitting
- Reaching
- Turning
- Pulling
- Pushing
- Driving

In short, all of the actions that are involved in everyday tasks. When we do them improperly, we're in trouble.

We should be taught as early as kindergarten that the body is a tool and that it has to be used in the right way. But since we're not, we lift, reach, push, and pull whatever way we feel like. By the time we're in our twenties and thirties, misuse starts to catch up with us. That's when we get the problems that are often attributed to disks (actually, most back pain cannot be related to disk changes), and we think we're doomed to be unlucky forever.

That's not true. *We can change our luck by using our bodies the way they were designed to be used.*

You've already made a start on changing things. Through body awareness, you've strengthened your kinetic memory.

Now you need to learn the physics of everyday movements.

Knowing these principles can get you into better shape. When you understand them, and use them along with other techniques, such as time management, you can control pain. You can do everything, from reaching for a box of files to picking up a package from the floor, in the way that is least likely to hurt you.

A Brief Primer on Body Physics
• • •

What I'm going to present now is mechanical information. It is basic. Yet you must understand it, because later on I'm going to show you how you can use it to keep pain out of your day.

The first lesson concerns that centerpiece of your anatomy: the spine.

The spine consists of vertebrae (chunks of bone) separated by disks (flat, fluid-filled pieces of cartilage), which act as "shock absorbers," easing the impact of the body's weight and allowing it to bend and to move. The spine is surrounded by layers of powerful muscles that hold the body erect.

To keep your spine and surrounding muscles healthy, you have first to realize their importance as the guardians of a pain-free life. Then you have to imagine them as your partners asking for help: "Take care of us, pal, so that we can take care of you."

Easy enough, you may think. But are you doing that right now? Which of the following statements apply to you?

- I sit for hours at a time without getting up.
- I slump forward or slouch backward when I stand, sit, or walk.
- I bend over repetitively in my work.
- I twist my body often in my movements.
- I repetitively reach up for things.
- I lift without bending my knees.
- I sleep on a soft mattress or sofa.

If you have any of these habits, you are putting stress on your spine and back muscles. If you have most of them, you are consistently misusing your body. That means your muscles have to work harder than they should, thus giving pain an opportunity to move in.

At this point you have to decide whether you want to do the work of replacing these unfortunate habits with better ways of doing things. If you *choose* to work on body physics, also called body mechanics, you have to ask yourself: What do my spine and back muscles want?

What Your Body Would Tell You

• • •

The first thing your body demands is good posture. Now some people think good posture means standing at attention. Wrong. Standing that way makes pain worse because your muscles become tense.

Good posture, as you learned when we discussed body awareness, means standing with your back straight, knees slightly bent, head up, chin in, and pelvis held straight. Your ears should be lined up with your shoulders. You are both aligned *and* comfortable.

A good way to get in touch with this posture is to lie on your back on the floor and align your body, as you do in the first body awareness movement. Then try to translate that feeling of being straight and wide into your stand-up posture.

Once you have established the correct posture, you're ready to move on to learning the basics of body mechanics.

Volumes have been written on this subject, but a lot of what you really need to know can be covered in one chapter. The principles are really all about doing right by your spine and back muscles.

In fact, a good way to think of them is as a "12-Step" program to keep your spine and back muscles happy:

STANDING 1. *Shift your weight frequently if you have to stand for a long time.* Whenever possible, put one foot up on a bar, box, or ledge. At a checkout counter, for example, you can rest your foot on the lower rung of the shopping cart. Alternate feet. Always avoid strain by wearing well-cushioned, low-heeled shoes.

SITTING 2. *Sit on a straight, hard chair that supports your back.* Your knees should be level with your hips, with your feet resting comfortably on the floor. Don't lean forward. To prevent slouching, tighten the muscles of your abdomen and lower back. For extra support, put a rolled-up towel or a lumbar pillow in the small of your back. Use a footrest to relieve pressure on your back. To get out of the chair, shift your weight forward, put one foot in front of the other, and get up.

SITTING 3. *Change positions frequently if you have to sit for a long time.* Shift your weight on the chair, cross your legs, or—better yet—get up occasionally and take a walk. If you can do a job standing up, such as dictating a letter or talking on the phone, do so. Or alternate between sitting down and standing up. Another possibility: Lie flat on your stomach with two pillows, one on top of the other, under your hips and another pillow under your shins.

BENDING 4. *Stand up—don't bend over—while doing a task,* such as brushing your teeth, for example, or washing a dish. Concentrate on keeping your back straight, your knees slightly bent, and your eyes looking straight ahead.

LIFTING 5. *If you have to lift something, bend with your knees and hips, not your back.* Squat down or go down on one knee, bring the object close to the front of your body, and lift, so that your legs, not your back, do the work. For example, to pick up a basket of laundry, bend down on one knee, move the basket close, and pick it up.

LIFTING 6. *Keep the weights you lift as light as possible.* Separate a load of wet laundry into several piles and lift one at a time. Break down a pile of documents into several piles and lift one at a time.

LIFTING 7. *Don't lift anything that's too heavy for you to handle.* Ask for help, wait for help, hire help—or walk away.

TURNING 8. *Pivot instead of twisting.* If you turn without moving your feet and hips, you're likely to twist your back, particularly if you're carrying something heavy. Instead, pivot—point one foot in the direction in which you want to go and let your whole body follow it around.

REACHING 9. *Don't stretch to get something that is out of reach.* Use a stool or ladder to get close to the item you want. As you lift, breathe out, thereby adding support to your back by tightening your abdominal muscles.

PUSHING 10. *Push an object using your legs for power, rather than pulling, whenever you can.* If you must pull, keep your feet apart and your knees bent and somewhat apart, and let your legs do most of the work.

CARRYING 11. *Carry packages and other heavy objects up close to the front of your body.* Carrying shopping bags by the handles weighs down your shoulders and may strain your back.

DRIVING 12. *Position the seat close to the pedals.* Also position it so that your knees are level with your hips and you have easy visibility without straining your neck and arms. When driving long distances, stop the car at least every thirty minutes and shift position or, even better, walk around the car and limber up.

Those are the basics. Of course, principles are easy enough to read about, but they are difficult to internalize unless you can see yourself or somebody else using them.

So let's create a scenario. Let's imagine that Lou Kostovich, the stock analyst I introduced you to earlier, has made plans to take a supply of tools to his boat on a Saturday morning so that he can repair a few things.

The night before, Lou sets the alarm clock so that he will wake up in plenty of time to do what he needs to do *slowly.*

He knows that HASTE = WRONG MOVEMENTS = PAIN.

As he dresses, Lou employs a few tricks he has learned to make the task more pain free. He lies down on the bed, for example, to put on his trousers, so that he doesn't have to bend over. To tie his shoelace, he puts his foot up on a chair, so he doesn't have to bend down to the floor.

When Lou gets downstairs to the kitchen, he discovers that his favorite breakfast cereal, which he usually keeps where he can reach it easily, has been put away in the cupboard. Although he could reach for the box, Lou remembers the "don't stretch" rule. Instead he stands on a stepladder to get the box.

Lou then goes to the basement to get the tools, which are in a box on a bottom cabinet shelf. Lou knows that the box is fairly heavy, so he gets two empty boxes. Then he squats down—bends with his knees and hips—and redistributes the tools so that he has three fairly light boxes. He lifts each box from a squatting position, after bringing it close to the front of his body. To turn around while carrying a box, Lou pivots.

While putting each box in the trunk of his car, Lou rests one foot on the bumper. This alleviates pressure on his lower spine.

As he opens the car door, Lou stands straight, with one foot slightly in front of the other and his knees slightly bent. In this position the weight of the car door will not push him backward as it swings open.

To get in, Lou backs through the door, sits down, and turns his body while lifting both feet in. He adjusts the seat so that his feet are close to the pedals and his knees level with his hips. He can now hold the steering wheel without straining his neck, shoulders, arms, and legs. For extra support, Lou uses a backrest. (The car, by the way, has an automatic shift, power steering, and power brakes.)

Lou knows that sitting is the least comfortable position for a person with low back pain. He also knows how long he can drive before he starts to feel discomfort.

Before he reaches his limit, Lou pulls over to a rest area. He gets out of the car and takes a brief walk. If Lou had been caught in a traffic jam and unable to move the car, he could have turned off the motor and adjusted his position on the seat several times.

When he arrives at the marina, Lou gets out of the car the same way he got in. He opens the trunk while standing straight with his knees slightly bent. Bending over would have strained his back.

Fortunately Lou's boat is moored fairly near the entrance to the marina, so he doesn't have far to carry the boxes. If the boat had been farther away, Lou would have asked for help, even though he hates having to do that. It's better, though, than overdoing and winding up in pain.

By the time Lou completes his morning's activities, he still feels comfortable and energetic. He is ready for the rest of the day.

Putting Your Mind Behind the Mechanics
• • •

Lou Kostovich's morning worked because *he* worked at it. As you can see by reading about the steps he took, body mechanics is a tradeoff. You trade the inconvenience of having to think about what you are doing for doing things in a way that doesn't hurt.

There's another point you may have realized, too: *Body mechanics is just as much a matter of attitude as it is physics.*

Though your body is a "machine" of sorts, it's run by your thoughts and your emotions. Notice we're back to that mind-body connection again. The truth is, you can't make body mechanics, or anything else in this program, work for you without putting your heart and mind behind it.

Your heart has to believe it has found a better way. Your mind has to struggle to overcome habit.

And habit is a very powerful force. Even as we understand that bending over or stretching to reach an object will cause us pain, we continue to do it. Even as we realize that groaning does nothing to reduce our pain, we continue to do it. Isn't that remarkable? Habit feels comfortable. It feels safe, *even as it hurts.*

Of course, poor habits are reinforced by thoughts, such as

- My body *should* be able to work the way I want it to.
- I *have to* do things the way I'm used to doing them.
- Poor me, I'm in so much pain. How can I be expected to learn something new?

So to succeed at body mechanics, you have to deal with such thoughts. And you also have to confront other attitudes that keep old habits in place. Here are some examples:

❑ **Embarrassment.** "How can I stop the car, get out, and walk around whenever I'm driving my friends someplace? I'd feel like a real jerk." This question came from Henry Carlson, the former construction worker I introduced you to in earlier chapters. I told Henry this:

Embarrassment comes from comparing what you are doing with what you think of as "normal." There really is no such thing. We must each do what is appropriate for us at the moment. If you fail to move in the way that is best for you, no matter how it looks to others, you will pay with pain, and indirectly those close to you will pay, too. Remember, coping is always better than remaining disabled.

❑ **Impatience.** "It takes too long to learn this stuff" is a comment I sometimes hear, particularly from people with many demands on their time. Of course, these are the very people who need to slow down and take the time to do things right. If you tend to be impatient, remember this—you have to choose between spending time on body mechanics or spending time in bed in pain. You don't get anything for nothing.

❑ **"I can't."** This is an attitude that has come up frequently in this book, and, as you know, it is a real killer. It is the giver-upper. It is the door closer. So you have to ask yourself: What is stopping me? Most often, you'll find that "I can't" really means "I won't": "I won't commit myself to learning different ways of thinking and acting so that I can take my life back from pain." "I won't" is a choice, but you can make a different choice by turning "I won't" into "I will."

Whenever you are faced with an everyday task you think you cannot do, you have to think instead, What can I do to solve this problem? This is the advice that Jane Prawda, the occupational therapist I mentioned in the previous chapter, gives to our patients:

If you are flexible, there is almost always a solution, and often there is more than one solution.

For example, in the chapter on time management, Rita Dawson, a schoolteacher, discovered that she could sit at her desk and mark papers more easily if she established a time baseline for performing this activity. But she also learned that she could expand the baseline by using several body mechanics techniques. For example, Rita could work on the task longer if she

- shifted her position on the chair frequently.
- took occasional walks.
- stood up to mark the papers.
- lay flat on her stomach to mark the papers.

By using *all* of these techniques, Rita became more comfortable with a job that had once been difficult. Most important, she was not embarrassed to be seen doing any of these things or impatient about remembering to do them. Rita knew that the only important thing was solving the problem.

You have to be thinking of solutions all the time, and you have to accept the solutions you learn—or invent—as normal for you. Never mind that other people may think them strange.

For example, let's imagine that you have given up on going to the supermarket because you find it painful to bend over to put things into the shopping cart or to take them out at the checkout counter. Here's a solution that Jane Prawda came up with: Place one or two shopping baskets upside down in the cart so that they create a kind of "shelf" that is easy to reach. This construction may look peculiar, but *ease is the only thing that counts.*

Or let's say that you find making a bed painful because you've been bending over to tuck in the sheet and blanket. Consider these two solutions:

1. Bend down on one knee at each corner to do the tucking.

2. Lie on your stomach on the bed to reach each corner to do the tucking.

The trick is to come up with an answer that's feasible for any given task.

For example, there are many adaptive aids you can buy that help with everyday activities. There are mechanical reachers so you don't have to stretch to get something down from a shelf; long-handled brushes for cleaning and bathing; wrist rests for extended work on a computer; twisting devices for opening jars and bottles; sock aids that make it easier to put on socks and pull them up; hooks for buttoning clothing; elastic shoelaces so you don't have to tie your shoes; and so forth. The number of items is almost endless, so it's worthwhile looking through the catalogs published by the companies that make them. Three useful names and addresses in this regard are Fred Sammons, Inc., "Enrichments," P.O. Box 579, Hinsdale, Ill. 60521, telephone: 1–800–323–5547; Independent Living Aids, Inc., 27 East Mall, Plainview, N.Y. 11803, telephone: 1–800–537–2118; and AliMed (office and workstation equipment), 297 High Street, Dedham, Mass. 02026–9135, telephone: 1–800–225–2610.

Remember that finding solutions to problems does not necessarily mean finding perfection. You may not be able to make a bed that could pass an army inspection. Yet you *will* be able to make a bed and make it without hurting yourself. This is where your sense of achievement should lie.

Whenever you plan what to do to accomplish a task, you also have to plan what will satisfy you. And satisfaction lies in

- being more free of pain.
- solving a problem.
- using a technique that will make you function better.

In short, satisfaction is obtained by concentrating on the process rather than on the results. When you think this way, you're certain to get the most out of body mechanics.

Ouch! When You Forget

• • •

There are moments when the principles of body mechanics fly out the window. You're busy at your desk when a paper falls to the floor. You're pressed for time, so without thinking you bend over to pick it up, rather than getting up from the chair and kneeling down on one knee. Or you get a phone call while your hands are busy with something you can't stop doing, so you twist your neck and hunch your shoulder to hold the receiver. Later on you find yourself in pain.

Almost everyone with CPS has noted that it's the little things that can mess you up, particularly when you are under stress. So it's during those stressful times that you have to say to yourself, Stand back, take a deep breath, practice your relaxation, slow down. As we learned from Lou Kostovich's example, slowing yourself down gives you time to remember to use your body as a tool.

But no one is perfect, and you'll forget sometimes. When that happens, don't come down on yourself too hard. Self-blame opens the door to catastrophizing and all the nasty things that follow. Tell yourself, I messed up—so what? And begin again.

It's easier to do your best when your home and work environments are set up to prevent the need for awkward, damaging movements. In fact, it's important to try to avoid making any unnecesssary, troublesome movements. The following steps can go a long way toward achieving this form of energy conservation:

❑ *Have the basics within easy reach.* Items you use every day, whether in your bedroom, bathroom, kitchen, office, or any other place, should be where you can get at them without stretching, bending, or climbing. In an office, for example, this may mean putting the most frequently used files in a middle drawer rather than in the top or bottom ones.

❑ *Say good-bye to clutter.* Pain becomes exacerbated when people have to lift and move piles of papers, clothing, and other items to reach what they really want. Pare "your stuff" down to things that you really use.

❑ *Get the height right.* Be sure that your desk chair is high enough to allow your bent elbows to rest comfortably on the desk. If you work on a computer, your hands should be lower than your elbows when your fingers are on the keyboard. The monitor should be directly above the keyboard, so that you don't have to strain your neck to see it.

❑ *Go light.* Look for the appliances and accessories that weigh the least. You want the lightest steam iron, lawn mower, vacuum cleaner, briefcase, laptop computer, and so on.

❑ *Use wheels.* Whenever possible, *roll* objects you have to move instead of carrying or pushing them. Wheeled carts, for example, can be used not only in the laundry room, but also in your office, basement workshop, and, particularly, the kitchen.

❑ *Ask for help.* You can't always go it alone when performing tasks. Get the assistance you need from family and friends.

Remember, too, that a steady supply of energy is necessary to do the tasks you have to do. Exercising, giving up narcotic drugs, getting a good night's sleep, managing your time properly, managing your body—these accomplishments charge your batteries. But there's yet another energy source to be tapped: eating in a way that fights pain.

STEP *11*

Escaping the Food Paradox

Since you developed chronic pain, you may have found yourself becoming more and more dependent on food, particularly junk food. I've found that weight gains of anywhere from twenty to forty pounds aren't unusual for chronic pain patients.

Those pounds come on because you're convinced that eating makes you feel better. And although friends and family may look askance as you snack away, the truth is you're right. Food actually reduces your pain in a number of ways:

1. *Emotional comfort.* Junk foods, with their connotation of deserved self-indulgence, can provide relief from a depressing situation.

2. *Chemical changes.* Eating certain foods increases the amount of serotonin, the natural antidepressant, in the brain, and serotonin makes endorphins, the pain-fighting chemicals, effective. So you really may *feel less pain* when your mouth is full.

3. *Distraction.* Buying food, finding it when you want it, preparing it, or merely tearing open a wrapper diverts your attention from pain.

All of these factors can make chronic pain sufferers more vulnerable to overeating than other people. So much for the guilt you may have been feeling.

But you must be aware of the paradox at work here. The relief you get from food is only temporary. After that there's a reverse effect, and the ultimate price you pay is more pain.

Think about it. Each extra pound that you put on strains muscles that have already been weakened by disuse and tension. These are the parts of your body that need to be made stronger in order to fight pain. So overeating sabotages your major goal of getting better. It is actually an assault on your body, says Julie Weiner, who teaches nutrition in my program.

There's another problem, too, Ms. Weiner points out. When you become habituated to certain foods, particularly junk foods, they start to work like narcotic drugs. You find that you need to eat more and more of them to get that "feel good" feeling. In time, food, which has masqueraded as the great comforter, fails to deliver. Instead it generates guilt, increased muscular tension, and more pain.

If you're engaged in an ongoing struggle with the refrigerator, you may wonder if you have the mental stamina to manage pain and lose weight at the same time.

"Doesn't it sound as if I'd be undertaking too much?" asked Marnie Singer, one of my patients, when we discussed the issue of weight loss.

The answer is no, because losing weight, if it's necessary, *is* part of pain management. And the techniques in this program— exercise, relaxation, and a better knowledge of how to cope, for example—can make it easier to eat less. As you master these techniques and consume less, you realize that you don't need to rely on food to feel better, just as you didn't need to rely on narcotic drugs to feel better. As you get stronger mentally and physically, you want to create a body that matches the way you feel.

That makes *now* just about the best time to put a mental lock on the refrigerator door.

You don't need a lecture on nutrition in order to do that.

You've probably heard the basics often enough. What you do need is to understand the types of foods that encourage pain and those that can help to alleviate it. *In sum, you have to look at nutrition from a pain-fighting point of view.*

Eating Right for Pain Control

• • •

Here's what you have to do:

❑ **Get off the blood sugar roller coaster.** The kinds of foods that make you "feel good" are generally refined carbohydrates—such as candies, chocolate, pastries, and jams. When you consume these foods, particularly on an empty stomach, your blood sugar rises, and you get the "high" you crave. But the high stems from physiological changes similar to those induced by stress, including *increased muscular tension.*

And as the "high" turns into a crash—which happens fairly quickly—you get stuck with depression, weakened, painful muscles, and a load of calories you didn't need. The same cycle of highs, lows, and muscular tension, by the way, can result from the use of caffeine.

You can control blood sugar—*and* lose weight—by decreasing your intake of refined carbohydrates (such as pastries) and increasing complex carbohydrates (such as pasta), protein (such as fish, poultry, lean meats, soybean products, and legumes), and low-fat dairy products. Replace caffeine—it's found in coffee, tea, cocoa, chocolate, and many soft drinks—with decaffeinated beverages and herbal teas.

❑ **Throw out the fat.** Fat stokes the pain machine because, like sugars, it quickly piles on the pounds, making your muscles work harder. A portion of fat (such as a pat of butter) has twice the number of calories as an equal-weight portion of complex carbohydrates or protein. Also, fat and cholesterol are suspected culprits in heart disease and certain cancers.

Red meat, luncheon meats, whole-milk dairy products, chocolate, and tropical oils (such as coconut, palm, and palm kernel oil —the types of oils frequently found in potato chips, baked goods, and other "feel good" snacks) are all high in fat. Substitute chicken, turkey, legumes, nonfat or low-fat dairy products, and monounsaturated fats (olive, peanut, and canola oils). Get no more than 30 percent of your total calories from fats.

❏ **Restore the balance.** Again and again I've showed you how physical and mental balance can put the brakes on pain. *Nutritional balance can do the same thing.* So in addition to complex carbohydrates, low-fat protein, and low-fat dairy products, be sure to include plenty of fruits, green vegetables, and yellow vegetables in your diet. The more types of good-for-you foods you can learn to enjoy, the less tempted you will be by the other kinds. Finally, ensure balance by taking a daily vitamin and mineral supplement.

If You Have Migraines or Arthritis
· · ·

Many migraine sufferers have found that avoiding certain foods and chemicals may decrease the frequency and the intensity of their headaches. Such foods include bacon, caffeine, frankfurters, fresh-baked yeast products, luncheon meats, nuts, red wines, tobacco, and foods containing monosodium glutamate (MSG), which is found in Chinese food, meat tenderizers, and preservatives.

Some people with arthritis find that *eliminating* the nightshade vegetables—tomatoes and eggplant—from their diet seems to relieve pain, as does *adding* greater quantities of fish. The Omega 3 fatty acids, found in fish oils, have anti-inflammatory properties. They are also known to reduce cholesterol.

There may be other foods to which individual arthritics are sensitive. For example, you may notice that your stiffness is aggravated after you eat dairy products, wheat products, or some other category of food.

If you suspect that you have a food allergy, keep a diary of what you eat. See if there are any particular foods that seem to be associated with flare-ups. Cut them out of your diet for a while and see if things get better. Restore them to your diet and see if things get worse. If they do, you may have discovered the culprits.

New Ways of Eating
· · ·

Having the food facts is one thing. Making the changes you need to make is another, as anyone who has ever tried to lose weight knows.

Right now you've been using food inappropriately in an attempt to make yourself feel better. But when you eat this way, your emotions manage your stomach. The way to lose weight is to eat only when you are hungry. Just that—and nothing more.

"But I'm hungry all the time," Marnie Singer told me.

I explained to Marnie that what she felt was not hunger, but the urge to comfort herself with food.

The next time you think you *must* have something to eat—and you've eaten pretty recently—ask yourself, What is this really all about? Most likely you'll uncover feelings of nervousness, sadness, and the like.

As soon as you recognize your emotions, reach out for the self-talk techniques you have employed at other points in this program. Tell yourself: These feeling don't mean that I *have* to eat. I can stand the discomfort of waiting for a while.

Discomfort is not a pleasurable state, but it can be a highly productive one, because it allows you to learn to cope more effectively. Remember that it will pay off as you lose weight, feel better about yourself, and control your pain.

Even as you feel uncomfortable, there are several "tricks" you can use to control eating binges:

❑ **Keep a diary.** If you write down everything you eat for a week or two—and no cheating—you may be astonished by the quantities of food you consume. Just seeing it all on paper can bring home the point: I've got to stop this.

❑ *Shop with an eye on labels.* The ingredients in food products are listed in order of quantity. Avoid buying foods that have sugars, fats, and cholesterol on the top of the list. That way they won't be in the house when you're tempted to reach for them.

❑ *Make mealtimes flexible.* Three meals a day are important, but the hours at which you eat should not be engraved in stone. Overweight people eat when "it's time," whether they're hungry or not. Slim people wait until they're really hungry.

❑ *Leave the table before you feel full.* It takes food a half hour to get into your bloodstream and satiate your hunger. So you've probably eaten enough way before you usually stop.

❑ *Realize that low-calorie snacks don't cancel out the other kind.* It sounds weird, but I can't tell you how often I've heard this excuse, "Well, Doctor, I may snack on ice cream, but I snack on salads, too." Acceptable snacks, such as raw vegetables, vegetable juice, or a fat-free plain yogurt, are not antidotes for those that are full of sugars and fats.

❑ *Seek constructive support.* Any help you can get from family and friends is well worthwhile, *if* these people can help you stick to your goal. Avoid "friends" who ask solicitously why you're putting yourself through all this now, when you are in pain.

❑ *Try it for a week.* If the thought of a long-term commitment to losing weight frightens you, tell yourself that you're just putting your toe in the water. You can do all the things I've suggested for just one week, can't you?

Marnie Singer decided to follow this approach. She put away foodstuffs she didn't want to touch, purchased a week's worth of nutritional foods, including low-calorie snacks, and committed herself to eating only when she was hungry—for a week.

And though she felt the discomfort of not reaching for her

"comfort blanket," Marnie experienced less pain. The reason was that she had freed herself of the self-blame and self-loathing on which pain feeds.

By the time the week was over, Marnie realized that she had lost two pounds, developed a new attitude, and gotten back lost self-esteem. She was encouraged to keep going for another week and then another—until she knew that *she* was stronger than her food habit.

Other Habits That Have Got to Go
• • •

Smoking deprives the muscles of oxygen, thus increasing pain. It makes exercising more difficult, and as you know, it has many other health risks, too. Unfortunately it is one of the most difficult habits to give up.

But, believe it or not, you *can* cut out smoking even as you are losing weight and doing everything else you need to do to stop pain.

One of my patients eliminated smoking gradually, in a manner similar to the way he had eliminated his use of narcotic drugs. He restricted himself first to ten cigarettes a day (he locked up the rest), then to nine, eight, and so forth. Some people find that they are able to quit "cold turkey." Others join special programs. There are many methods, but the point is to find one that you feel comfortable with *now*, while you are energized to make your life better.

You have to evaluate your use of alcohol, too. Although alcohol can relieve pain and stress temporarily, it is a depressant, and when the initial effects wear off, it leaves you more depressed and anxious than you were when you picked up the glass.

Even so, alcohol, like food and cigarettes, can be quite tempting as a source of pain relief. That's why it's best to steer clear of it altogether and rely on techniques that *you* control in order to manage your pain.

If you're already fighting an alcohol dependency, you know

how much more difficult chronic pain can make the struggle. You need to keep up your contacts with Alcoholics Anonymous, a therapist, or whatever source of assistance you've been using, as you work on this program. At Lenox Hill I give patients who need them the locations of AA meetings in the area, so that they can attend while they are with us. It's tough enough to do everything you have to do in this program without having to cope alone with the torture of wanting to reach for a drink.

Self-help organizations, such as AA, encourage their members to examine subjects like feelings and relationships. And these topics are important for *any* person with chronic pain, because feelings are a component of the syndrome.

If you're not in touch with your feelings, and if your family relationships are not as healthy as they might be, the road to recovery can be blocked. But there are ways to remove those roadblocks and to make your life inestimably richer by doing so. This is what I am going to show you how to do next.

Getting Connected to Your Feelings

W hen I introduced you to this program, I told you that chronic pain was *garbage* in your mind in that it serves no purpose. But there's more to the garbage analogy, because chronic pain is also a kind of *dump*. Whatever is bothering you in life, whatever history you may be trying to escape, whatever emotions you don't want to deal with—they can get buried here.

So you have to think of your pain not only as a problem in its own right, but also as a stand-in for something else. That something else is your feelings.

When we are disconnected from our feelings, we cannot know, much less achieve, what we truly want in life. There's another danger, too. As you get totally absorbed in your pain—with feelings of anxiety, hopelessness, and despair about it—you fail to recognize that you also have affirmative feelings. Just as chronic pain takes over your day, it seems to overshadow your other emotions:

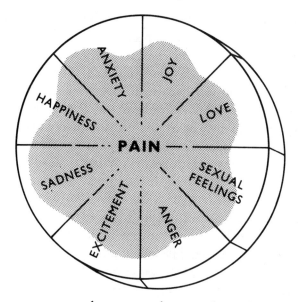

If you want to get better, you have to do an excavation job. You have to dig in order to find out what may be underneath it all, obscured by pain.

This is not easy to do because chronic pain is an acceptable excuse for *not* facing such feelings. Chronic pain may be uncomfortable, but it's safe, too, because it's considered a physical problem. Attributing your suffering to emotional difficulties may be harder to bear and less justifiable, both to yourself and to those around you.

So the excavating I'm asking you to do can be more of a challenge than anything else I've asked of you thus far. And I know my request can produce a "pull-back response" in your mind. You may get an urge to put down this book. You may decide, This talk of buried emotions can't possibly apply to me.

But please bear with me. Suppression is something that's fairly easy to spot in other people but quite difficult to see in ourselves.

Let me give you an extreme example, that of Shelley Menton, one of my patients.

Everyone—my staff, myself, and the other patients—could see that Shelley was a deeply unhappy person. She held us all at arm's length, refusing to let anyone break through her shell. Yet Shelley, a thirty-five-year-old computer specialist, insisted that there was nothing wrong except for the severe headaches she had been suffering *daily* since the age of six. Her childhood, Shelley reported, had been a happy one. It just "happened" that she had never wanted to make any friends or to allow anyone to get close to her. "It's better that way," she told me, since other people could not be trusted.

Shelley had experienced one romantic involvement, which ended when the young man left her. When I asked Shelley what she felt about that, she shrugged. "Nothing," she said. "I expected it."

Since the affair ended, Shelley's headaches had become even more intense and her social contacts more sparse. Still, Shelley declared that her life would be fine if only the headaches could be cured. Emotionally, she insisted, she was in top shape.

I have found that many of my patients get to know each other in group sessions and care about each other very much, and Shelley's group refused to stop reaching out to her. Everyone could see how miserable she was, *except Shelley herself.*

I finally confronted her: "You have to recognize that you have been sad and frightened for most of your life. All you have to do is look in the mirror. The muscles of your face are so constricted that they are frozen in place."

Shelley rummaged through her purse for a compact, looked in the mirror, and, for the first time in her life, was able to see the sad person everyone else confronted the first moment they met her. Only then was she able to begin to accept the help that my staff and I were offering her.

When Shelley Menton looked in the mirror and saw tense muscles, she was looking at the mechanism that kept her feelings under control. These muscles were like a very tight fist that kept something from escaping.

But as Shelley worked on her body awareness, relaxation practice, and the inner journey, she found that feelings started to emerge. *That's because relaxation releases the muscles, and as muscles are released, feelings and memories can get released, too.*

Not everyone has this experience, but many people do, sometimes in a very graphic fashion. Several years ago, for example, while lying on the floor doing a body awareness movement, a patient suddenly remembered having been sexually abused as a child. Even while she sobbed uncontrollably, she realized that something remarkable was happening to her body: her pain was starting to go away.

Usually memories and feelings come to the surface more gradually and less dramatically. Shelley, for example, reported her feelings only as "strange." Other people have described sensations as varied as "feeling sad," "being restless," "trembling," and "having a desire to cry."

These sensations are so unexpected—after all, relaxation is associated with pleasure—that people sometimes think something is wrong. "When I start to relax, a sad thought will appear, and I can't get it to go away," a patient told me with concern.

I explained to this man that his goal should not be to make the feeling go away. Instead he had to allow himself to experience it, even though he found it frightening.

If you are having sensations that seem unusual to you, don't pull back from them. "The heart has its reasons which reason knows nothing of," wrote the French philosopher Blaise Pascal. Being given the chance to uncover your heart's reasons is actually a great gift, a positive aspect of your chronic pain experience.

Many people go around half alive, caught in an emotional rut that they never try to analyze. But chronic pain, in a strange way, has forced introspection upon you. Pain, which laid you low, can actually be an opportunity to turn your life around, *if you have the courage to look at what is bothering you.*

Facing Your Feelings
. . .

As I stated earlier, chronic pain covers up other emotions, so you have to work on separating your newly emerging feelings from your reactions to pain.

The first step is to tolerate these feelings. Let them out. Allow yourself to cry if you feel like it.

The next step is to look within. For example, don't just recognize that you are feeling sad. Ask, What am I really sad about? Here are other types of questions you could ask yourself:

- What am I anxious about? Is there some situation that I am afraid to deal with?
- Am I involved in relationships that are unsatisfying or damaging to me?
- Do I have memories about my parents or my childhood that are upsetting to me?
- Do I conceal my emotional needs from my friends and family?
- Have I been pretending that certain problems aren't there?

These questions may seem strange to you if, like some people with CPS, you avoid recognizing that what's happening to you—or has happened to you—affects the way you feel. Such avoidance is like throwing away an emotional compass. It dooms you to being perpetually lost.

For example, the night before Arthur Brandt was to go home for the weekend after his first week in my program, he tossed and turned for hours. This surprised Arthur because he had been sleeping well for the first time in a long time after entering the hospital.

"I can't imagine why I couldn't sleep," Arthur remarked to me.

"Don't you think you might be anxious about going home and

losing the support you've been getting from the staff and the other patients?" I asked.

Arthur looked at me in amazement. He was so removed from his own feelings that it hadn't occurred to him to wonder why he might be having an anxiety response, such as sleeplessness, to a significant change in his circumstances.

So looking inside yourself, taking the trouble to make connections, can get you a lot closer to what's going on.

One way to make connections is to write down the feelings that emerge while you're doing a relaxation technique. Try to note everything you associate with the feeling—events that are happening currently and memories of the past. Also keep a pad on the night table so you can write down significant dreams. (This, along with your sleep diary, is one of the "permissible" reasons for writing at night.) Your dreams, by the way, can become quite vivid when you first start to use relaxation techniques, particularly the inner journey. These "loaded" dreams are a repository for feelings that are coming to the surface.

Thinking About What You Find
• • •

What kinds of things might you discover when you connect to your feelings?

- *Anger* about something in the past or present.
- *Disappointment* either in yourself, in someone you are close to, or in life itself.
- *Fear* of someone, a boss, for example, or a spouse, lover, or parent.
- *Anxiety* about becoming too close to someone you love.
- *Resentment* at being used by others or at having your needs unmet.
- *Distress* at sexual feelings that you find unacceptable.

Once you become aware of such feelings, you can *choose* to give yourself the courage to work at changing situations that may be inadvertently keeping you in the grip of CPS. If it turns out that pain was a convenient way of avoiding these problems, you will have removed a reason for your pain.

For example, let's consider a situation that faced Toni Romano, to whom I introduced you at the beginning of this book. I told you how Toni had always been the mainstay of her large, extended family, even though she was raising three children on her own. If there was trouble, Toni's siblings called her. If they were short of money, they called her. If their aged father had to be taken care of, they called her.

When Toni first started to do the relaxation practice, she found it hard to concentrate because a vision of storm clouds always intruded into the inviting beach scene that she was trying to create. At first this image frightened her. But as Toni stopped trying to push it away, she realized that the clouds represented her demanding family, always swooping down on her.

With awareness of the situation came the choice: What to do? She could continue to be "good old dependable Toni"—perfect daughter and sister—or she could opt to change things. Toni decided to get together with her siblings and, in a loving way, talk over the way she felt. (I'll tell you how Toni handled this discussion later on.) And although Toni's brothers and sisters were surprised, they agreed to try to do more for themselves. As the situation slowly changed, Toni's feelings of resentment began to diminish, as did her pain.

As Toni's case demonstrates, awareness can often allow you to deal with problems—stemming sometimes from the present, sometimes from the past—that have been hidden from you. But awareness can do something else as well. It can encourage you to see *what chronic pain has done to your relationships with family and friends.*

I don't have to tell you that chronic pain has long tentacles. Everyone within its range gets caught in its grasp, especially those nearest and dearest to you. As they struggle to help you, and also to help themselves, your family may react in ways that are damaging to your recovery. With the best of intentions, unhealthy family patterns and relationship patterns can grow up around chronic pain.

Here are two of the most common. Do either of them sound familiar?

• PATTERN ONE •
"Let Us Take Care of You, Dear."

Your family does almost everything for you so that you don't have to exert yourself and risk bringing on pain. If you groan or scrunch up your face, they ask, "What's wrong, dear?" If you look as if you might try doing something they think is too hard for you, they say, "*We'll* do that, dear." They don't seem to have much time for their own activities. Your needs take priority.

All you have to do is look around, see who's waiting on you currently, and ask, "While you're up, could you get me a Scotch?"

Though your family may sigh and groan a lot, just the way you do, they keep on doing *for* you.

So the upshot is: You get rewarded for being in pain.

This luxurious treatment is a gold mine for the needy part of you, which seems to want more and more. It's like sinking into a warm, cozy pit. But cozy though it may be, the price is high, because *you wind up with someone else living your life.*

Taking care of your daily needs—dressing, cooking, cleaning, shopping, going to work, taking out the garbage, putting up with hassles—this *is* life. When you don't do these things, *to the extent that you can,* it's hard to have integrity or self-esteem.

If you feel you're losing these qualities, ask yourself: Am I doing everything I'm capable of doing? Or have I slid into a comfortable, dependent situation?

If the latter is true, have a gentle talk with your family. Tell them, "I know you love me. But if you really want to help me, this is what you can do for me:

- Help me move *gradually* toward being more independent.
- Encourage me to keep doing the activities in my pain management program.
- Understand that I can exercise and do things in a *graded manner* without hurting myself.
- Try not to react to my pain behaviors. In fact, when you catch me at them, tell me they are inappropriate.
- Support me through setbacks.
- Don't agree with me when I tell you 'I can't.'
- Get yourself involved in other things besides me.
- Realize that the *less* compulsively you do things for me, the *more* you help me keep my commitment to getting better."

• PATTERN TWO •
"Why Don't You Just Grin and Bear It, Dear?"

Your family was once supportive, but now they don't seem to take your pain seriously. Whether they kiss you off with a kindly, "You're okay, honey," or a more severe, "Life is tough, why don't you just get on with it?" you feel as if no one understands. People listen to you less and less. In fact, they try to keep out of your way.

Some families are naturally uncommunicative, but that's not usually the reason they start leaving a CPS sufferer alone or giving him or her stiff-upper-lip advice. Most often these things happen when the family gets sick and tired of hearing about pain. *In short, the sufferer has become a drag.*

The more absorbed you become in your pain, the more you push other people away—just when you need them most. And although you feel abandoned, *you* may be the one who is actually abandoning others.

If you think you are very much alone, ask yourself: Is pain the *only* thing that I share with my family? Would I want to be close to someone who did nothing but think and talk about pain?

If you answered yes to the first question and no to the second, it's time to sit down with your family and have a gentle talk. Tell them, "I know you love me, and I'm sorry that we have moved away from each other. We can try to get close again, if you will do the following:

- Don't walk away from my pain behaviors. Instead, point them out to me. Ask me to stop.
- Encourage me to keep doing the activities in my pain management program.
- Help me to focus on other things besides my pain. Ask me to tell you at least one 'nonpain' story a day.
- Don't be afraid to talk about having fun in front of me. I want to share your experiences by hearing about them, even if I can't do everything you can do right now.
- Include me in making family plans and in performing family chores, *to the best of my ability.*
- Share your world with me, and I will find it easier to get back into that world."

The Beginning of Change
· · ·

The way to start altering unhealthy family patterns is to listen to what your family needs and to let your family know what you need.

To get your needs across, you have to be able to express yourself in a way that makes people respond to you, rather than infantilize you, get angry at you, or shut you out. In sum, you need to use assertive, *pain-relieving communication.*

Much has been written about assertiveness. *But it has not often been pointed out that failing to be assertive is related to chronic pain.*

"I've got a pain in my back," a patient once challenged me. "Where does not being assertive fit in?"

The answer, I told him, is that if you fail to tell people what you want, you become resentful, the tension in your muscles increases, and the pain in your back gets worse. On the other hand, if you make angry, aggressive demands in an effort to control others, the tension in your muscles increases, and the pain in your back gets worse. These two extremes—passivity and aggressiveness —get in the way of constructive, assertive behavior.

Two examples, concerning patients I mentioned earlier in this chapter, will demonstrate what I mean.

One afternoon, Arthur Brandt wanted to help his son, Ben, paint the porch. But Ben feared that the work would increase his father's pain. He discouraged his father from helping. Arthur knew that he couldn't do as much painting as he used to do, but he felt that he needed to do *as much as he could* in order to feel better about himself. Arthur wanted to tell his son this, but then he stopped himself. He thought: Ben's been doing so many things for me since I got sick. I depend on him. And he's been good to me. How can I get him upset? It will be better if I don't say anything.

When Arthur told me this story, he believed he had been assertive because he had handled the situation in the "only way possible." Actually, I pointed out, the situation didn't get handled at all, because the conflict hadn't been resolved. (The only discussion took place in Arthur's head.) In fact, Arthur's passivity made any interaction with his son impossible, and it served only to perpetuate his pain behaviors.

Shelley Menton informed me, when we discussed pain-relieving communication, that she had "no trouble being assertive" with her co-workers.

"What do you do?" I asked, knowing that Shelley could get quite angered by the amount of work that was routinely piled on her desk.

"I just take those papers and shove them back at them, or I pick up the phone and tell them where they can get off."

As Shelley recounted this, the muscles in her face became even tighter, and I could tell that her pain felt worse. Her style of talking to colleagues was like stoking up a pain machine. And Shelley's aggressiveness, like Arthur's passivity, failed to change the basic situation. Those papers kept on coming, as did the headaches.

Assertive, pain-relieving communication is quite different from passivity and aggressiveness. It is the only way of dealing with people that actually *solves problems and preserves relationships at the same time.* When you communicate in a pain-relieving manner, you try not to "beat" the other person, but to effect changes that are acceptable to both parties.

As you can imagine, this takes some work. Repressing what you really want or flying off the handle is a far easier course. To communicate your needs assertively, you have to *pay attention* to what you are doing. You have to

- make certain, in any given situation, that you're dealing with something that can actually be changed.
- clearly and calmly state your needs and preferences.
- listen to the other person's needs and preferences in a sympathetic manner.
- present your arguments in a diplomatic way.
- demonstrate confidence in your own opinions.
- show that you care about the other person's opinions.
- refuse to let yourself be stepped on.
- avoid behaving angrily or judgmentally.
- steer clear of bullying, threatening, and name calling.

Why does communicating in this manner prevent an increase in pain?

For one thing, it is a *caring* form of talking with people, and therefore it avoids the anxiety and guilt that we frequently experience when we lack compassion in dealing with others. These emotions lead to muscular tension—and pain.

If your natural tendency is to be aggressive, assertive communication relieves you of the pain-provoking belief that you "should" be able to control other people by making demands. If your natural tendency is to be passive, it relieves you of the pain-provoking belief that the other person "should" understand you without your having to say what you want. Finally, assertiveness keeps you in balance—*and balance is always an effective means of controlling pain and suffering.*

A Pain-relieving Family Conference
· · ·

I said that assertive communication requires you to pay attention, to care about others, and to keep conflict at a minimum. Let me show you what can be achieved when you do these things.

When Toni Romano decided to tell her siblings that she needed them to do more for themselves, her first consideration was: Am I asking something of them that they can do? The answer was yes, since all were adults with a reasonable level of maturity.

Toni invited her family over so that they could chat in the comfort of her living room. In a pleasant manner, she gave them her view of the situation. She said, "You all know that I've been suffering from chronic pain for many years. Now I've learned some ways of making my pain better. One thing that would help me, I realize, would be for you to take over more of the family responsibilities I've been handling. Let's talk about how we can manage that."

This statement made the problem a group problem, which could be solved if everyone worked together.

Toni's siblings were surprised by her request. They insisted, somewhat angrily at first, that they hadn't been imposing on her at all. (After all, it's always difficult to break established patterns.)

Toni didn't respond to their anger. She listened patiently, nodded frequently, and repeated back what they had told her, indicating that she understood what they *thought* had been happening.

Then she went on to give them specific examples of occasions where she believed they had asked for her help unnecessarily. She told them how overburdened these incidents had made her feel.

She wasn't judgmental. She simply asked them to think about ways they might have managed by themselves.

As her brothers and sisters listened to Toni, they began to realize how much of her time they had taken up and how unaware they had been of her feelings. They started to talk about how things might be handled differently in the future. In the course of the discussion, several siblings expressed anxiety at the thought of losing Toni's support, and Toni saw that they hadn't merely been imposing on her; they depended on her emotionally.

The discussion ended with Toni's siblings promising to try to do more for themselves and with Toni promising to still be there for them, but in a more limited manner. *Toni wound up with some of what she needed, and her siblings wound up with some of what they needed.* Most important, relationships were enriched, because buried feelings on both sides had been brought to the surface.

I have to tell you that pain-relieving communication is always a work in progress. It's something you have to strive for, and no one, not even the great gurus, achieves perfection at it. What's more, it doesn't get you what you want all of the time. But even when it doesn't, you'll learn a lot, because when you reveal your frustrations and disappointments, so will the individual you are talking with—sometimes to your displeasure but ultimately to your mutual benefit.

Another bonus of this communication style is that it enables you to feel good about asking for what you want. *For a person with CPS, that's imperative because you have to make your needs known in order to get back into life.* When you commit yourself to being assertive, you learn that it's usually possible to create options that can help you.

Arthur Brandt, for example, had given up playing the drum in the community marching band he'd belonged to for fifteen years. "I love it, but the drum's too heavy to carry, so that's the end of that," he told me.

But as he understood the importance of assertiveness, Arthur began to think of how he could manage to keep doing something he loved. He figured out several alternatives, among them to:

- persuade the band director to get him a stand on wheels to carry the drum.
- get someone else to agree to carry the drum for him.
- ask the director to buy a lighter drum for him to use.

Even though Arthur didn't want to ask for help or stand out from the other band members, he realized that demonstrating assertive behavior would be good for him. He had to put one fact first: *He wanted to play the drum.* That meant he couldn't "cop out" on taking action. He had to think, *I want something. I have choices. I don't have to be a victim.*

It was tough to do, but Arthur approached the band director, telling the man, who was now without a drummer, "Let's talk about how we can solve both our problems."

I'm glad to tell you that Arthur's band purchased a lighter, smaller drum for him. But no one would have thought of this move if Arthur hadn't made the suggestion himself. And even if he had been turned down, Arthur would have discovered that simply having the courage to speak up diminished his suffering.

When You Need to Get Help

. . .

Many times, like Arthur and Toni, you can work toward solving a problem on your own. But some family relationships are too troubled, and some feelings are too distressing, for you to deal with by yourself. This is especially true if you have difficulty in recognizing your feelings or in accepting them.

If you realize that your relationships with family and friends are unsatisfactory, or if you find yourself boxed in by unsettling emotions that you don't understand, you should consider getting help from a therapist.

Now I know that the mere mention of therapy can be a red flag for someone who suffers from chronic pain. After all, the recommendation "*You* should see a psychiatrist" may have been made to you in the past in a negative way. Perhaps you thought the statement implied that you were mentally ill.

But I think you know by now that I am not implying anything like that. Chronic pain is not a "mental problem." But chronic pain can appear to be an untreatable curse *unless* you deal with the emotional components of your suffering. When the lid on your feelings is very tight, you may need some assistance taking it off. Why deny yourself the chance to get help from professionals experienced in lid removal?

Therapists are trained to help you tolerate the discomfort of looking at thoughts and feelings that you find unacceptable. They can assist in putting pieces together and in developing choices that you may not have considered.

So if you have a prejudice against therapy, try to put it aside. Think of therapy as an opportunity to learn to function better—and remember that nothing is more important than reaching that goal.

It's best to select a therapist who is experienced in working with chronic pain patients. Such therapists generally practice cognitive behavior therapy, the type that underlies many of the principles in this book. Cognitive behavior therapy encourages you to function as well as you can, even as you uncover the reasons for your feelings and work toward solutions for your problems. It doesn't put real life on "hold" while you try to get to the bottom of things. It *is* real life.

A final thought about therapy: Life is constructed so that there is only one game in town. It is called reality, and anything we can do to help ourselves deal with reality is a blessing. In fact, it's a privilege to be able to work on getting to know yourself better, and the rewards can be great.

The subject of rewards brings us back to the beginning of this book, when I introduced you to my program. I told you then that managing pain required hard work, but that you would be amply rewarded for it. I hope that you have already begun to experience these dividends. If not, be assured that they will come.

Remember, you are just at the beginning. There is no limit to how much better you can feel and to how much more you can accomplish. Don't dwell on the past. You are on your way to having the tomorrows you want.

Putting It All Together

You've got the techniques, you've got the motivation, and you know you have the power to move pain to the periphery of your day.

But you may need some assistance in visualizing how everything you've learned can work together.

It can help, I think, to look at one day in the life of a former CPS sufferer. The example I'll use is that of Lou Kostovich, the stock analyst I introduced to you when we talked about the physics of movement.

It's 6:30 A.M., and Lou's alarm clock has just gone off. Today there's an important meeting coming up at work. Lou expects some conflict, with himself on one side and some high-powered opponents on the other.

Knowing that the meeting could be a pain-activating trigger, Lou prepared for it last night by doing an inner journey in which he saw two divided sections of a forest growing together, a metaphor for difficulties being resolved. Lou also thought about his goals for the meeting and visualized himself achieving them in an effective manner.

Finally, Lou planned how he would use his time for the day. He scheduled three "musts"—the meeting, the completion of a report, and a telephone conference relating to a new project. Also on Lou's agenda are such want-tos as lunch with an old friend and attending a concert with his wife, Melanie.

Lou gets out of bed, feeling a bit stiff and achy, but he is thinking, I feel some pain. That's okay. I can deal with it. He does his "holy half hour" of exercises. Since Lou has allowed plenty of time to get ready for work, he can do the exercises slowly and carefully, without feeling pressured.

Lou showers and dresses, also slowly, so that he can think about pulling on his pants, putting on socks, and tying his shoes in ways that do not cause pain. He goes into the kitchen, where he and Melanie prepare breakfast together. All of the ingredients Lou needs are kept on a low shelf, so he can get at them without having to reach up. Lou is on a diet, cutting back on fat and cholesterol and trying to lose the weight he put on when he was a "pain person." Lou doesn't care for dieting, but he thinks, I can stand the discomfort of giving up some foods I like, because I know that losing weight will ease my pain.

As the Kostoviches enjoy breakfast, Lou avoids talking about his pain. Instead he and Melanie discuss how much they are looking forward to the concert.

Lou has a heavy pile of papers to take to the office for the meeting, so he divides them into two separate briefcases. He will carry one case in each hand.

Before Lou starts his car, he does a relaxation practice, since he anticipates that the morning traffic jam might make him tense.

Today the jam turns out to be worse than usual. Several drivers are honking their horns and behaving in a totally brainless fashion, but Lou restrains himself from feeling angry. I wish they wouldn't be such jerks, he thinks, but that's the way it is. People do what they want to do, not what I'd like them to do.

Since it looks as if he'll be stuck for some time, Lou does a full relaxation practice. Then he shifts his position a few times. Finally, to distract himself, he listens to an audiotape of a recent best-seller. He thinks of that cloak of comfort Dr. Douglas talks about and tries to visualize the cloak wrapping itself around him now.

The traffic jam eases, and a short while later Lou arrives at his office. He seats himself on his comfortable desk chair and sips a cup of caffeine-free coffee. He uses a special pillow to support his back, and he keeps a footrest near the desk, too.

Lou works on completing the report. His secretary has placed the files he needs on the front of the desk so that he doesn't have to reach for them.

The big meeting is scheduled for ten-thirty. As the time approaches, Lou feels his palms starting to get cold and clammy. He uses his relaxation technique. Then he visualizes himself in the meeting, as he did the night before, presenting his arguments in a persuasive way. Lou tells himself that he can only do his best. He cannot make things turn out perfectly.

At the actual meeting, Lou enumerates his points in an assertive manner. He is respectful of the opposing viewpoint, but he refuses to let himself be bullied by one colleague, whose smooth tone can't hide the fact that he is trying to stick a knife into Lou.

Lou finds that diaphragmatic breathing, which he has been doing consistently, relaxes him. He thinks, I wish this guy wouldn't be such a creep, but I can't control what other people do. I can only point out the discrepancies in what he's saying.

About half an hour into the meeting, Lou gets up from his chair and walks around the room. Lou has informed his colleagues of the need for these "breaks" from sitting, and now they scarcely notice them.

Negotiations continue, and some important points are settled, but the meeting ends, to Lou's frustration, with the major decision being held off for another week. Well, he thinks, I managed to get some of what I wanted. And I kept my pain at a minimum. Pretty good, all in all. I can stand to wait a while longer for the final outcome.

At lunch, Lou sticks to his diet. He has deliberately selected a restaurant that specializes in a low-fat menu, to make food selection easier. Although Lou has noticed a slight increase in pain as a result of the morning's meeting, he is able to distract himself by getting involved in his friend's stories of a recent Caribbean vacation.

He returns to the office feeling refreshed, but in the afternoon a crisis develops. A package of material, which Lou sent by overnight express the day before, has apparently failed to arrive at the hotel where it's needed for an important presentation. Lou's boss looks highly annoyed.

Lou starts to think, Oh, my God, I'm going to lose my job. He's put up with my pain problem long enough, and now this. I've had it. Then he breathes deeply, relaxes, and reflects: I'm having catastrophic thoughts. The problem isn't my boss, but the lost package. I'll put my energy into solving the real problem.

Lou assembles replacement copies of some of the material that he shipped. Perhaps it can be faxed. In the meantime, his secretary discovers, after a fractured conversation with a hotel employee who doesn't speak much English, that the package has been located, buried under some convention supplies. It will be delivered at once, or at least that's what she understands the man to say.

Now that the crisis appears to be over, Lou and his secretary have a good laugh over the garbled conversation. The laughter distracts Lou from the pain that has been building up.

Lou asks his secretary to cancel the telephone conference, deciding that he needs to work on something less stressful during the afternoon. He closes the door to his office and reviews the rest of his report, while lying flat on his stomach on the floor, with pillows under his hips and shins. When he's finished with the report, Lou does three body awareness movements and then stands up, feeling more relaxed.

Later on, after a dinner out, Lou and Melanie attend the concert. They stay for only the first half, as they had planned, since Lou is not yet ready to sit for an extended period of time. The Lou with CPS would have resented missing out on part of a concert, but the recovering Lou is willing to get enjoyment out of what is feasible for him.

On the way home, the Kostoviches talk about what happened during the day. Lou tells Melanie that he feels proud of his performance during the meeting. He goes on to amuse her with the story of the lost package. He refrains from talking about any pain he might feel. In spite of its many stresses, this has been a *good* day.

Later that night Lou and Melanie make love, something they had stopped doing when Lou was totally focused on his pain. They use the side position, in which both partners face each other. This position is comfortable when a man has back pain, as it allows the woman to do most of the hip movement.

A few hours later, when Lou wakes up, he does an inner journey to help him fall back to sleep. On the journey he sees a beautiful Indian princess coming toward him through the forest and guiding him toward a river of gold. Lou realizes that the princess is Melanie. When he returns from the journey, the house seems to be full of love.

What Happens Next?

Pain management, once successfully achieved, is a lifelong commitment that demands strict fidelity. You can never be "too bored," "too tired," or "feeling too good" to ignore its requirements. But it's not likely, once you have come this far, that you will be tempted to slough off. If you've been practicing the program faithfully, you've probably found that its tenets have become ingrained in you, rather like a dancer's need to limber up before going to work.

However, if you ever go through a period when events prevent you from paying close attention to the program, and you need some extra impetus to get back into it, you may want to consider adding the following two resources. I didn't include them in this book (although I use them at Lenox Hill), because you need professional help to do them.

One is biofeedback. In this procedure, a trained professional hooks you up to a device with a monitor that measures the stress levels in various parts of your body. With the therapist's help, you are able to observe that you can lower those levels by practicing relaxation techniques. So the machine provides proof positive that relaxation works. But it also tunes you in to your body quite subtly so that you can see exactly what is required to alter your particular physiology. This knowledge increases your ability to practice relaxation at home.

Another procedure, TENS (transcutaneous electrical nerve stimulation), is based on the theory that a small electrical current applied to nerve endings may block pain. This is done by means of electrodes, placed on the pain sites and connected to a small machine that can be worn on your belt. Some people find that TENS gives them an additional means of fighting pain, although a disadvantage is that it requires dependency on a machine. TENS can also be less effective as time goes on.

You may have had some thoughts about enrolling in a pain management program yourself. Although there are over 1,500 such programs in the country, the Commission on the Accreditation of Rehabilitation Facilities (CARF) accredits only about 135 of them, my own included. To find out about accredited programs in your area, contact the commission at 101 No. Wilmot Rd., Suite 500, Tucson, Ariz. 85711. Telephone: 1–800–444–8991. To receive information about my program, send a self-addressed, stamped envelope to the New York Pain Treatment Program, Lenox Hill Hospital, 130 E. 77th St., New York, N.Y. 10021, or phone 1-800-548-3242.

As you may have surmised, there can be vast differences among programs. Some concentrate only on procedures, such as injections of steroids or nerve blocks. Others focus totally on exercises. But doing just one thing is like trying to bake a cake using only one ingredient. It simply doesn't come out right.

You need the type of multifaceted approach that you have been given in this book, which means the program has to have a team: a physician, psychologists, physical therapists, biofeedback specialists, occupational therapists, and nurses who will work closely with you on everything from exercising to the inner healing of the mind.

Before you enroll in any program, question the director as closely as he or she is questioning you. Try to get an idea of the program's scope, how long it has been in existence, and how many patients it has served. Ask for the names of former patients you can talk with. And, if possible, see if you can observe the facility.

Make it a point to meet several of the staff people you will be working with. Ask yourself whether you feel comfortable with them and whether they seem to be empathetic toward your situation. If you don't sense a "good fit," the program is not likely to work for you, and you should look elsewhere.

If you're not interested in an actual program, but feel you need help in continuing to practice what you've learned from this book, you may benefit from joining a support group. Nobody knows what you've been going through—and what you need to do now—better than the people you'll meet in these groups.

There are two major national support groups.

The American Chronic Pain Association has 650 self-help chapters in the United States and abroad. Each group is led by a person with chronic pain. Address: P.O. Box 850, Rocklin, Calif. 95677. Telephone: 1-916-632-0922.

The National Chronic Pain Outreach Association, Inc. (NCPOA), maintains a computerized registry of support groups in the United States and Canada. Send a number 10 self-addressed, stamped envelope for information. Address: 7979 Old Georgetown Rd., Suite 100, Bethesda, Md. 20814-2429. Telephone: 1-301-652-4948.

A support group that meets regularly can be an important element in creating structure in your life. But, as you know, you also need to work hard at creating that structure yourself, particularly if you are no longer working.

If that's the case, and you will not be able to return to your old job at some point, you must go about getting retrained for a new type of employment, something that is feasible in terms of your present physical condition.

My program, like other comprehensive pain management programs, links patients to organizations that can provide vocational counseling. Your state vocational rehabilitation agency, for example, can give you guidance in this regard.

Your local community college can also be an invaluable resource for retraining. Many of these colleges have large adult student populations, programs designed for them, and counselors on hand to assist with their vocational needs. If you feel anxious about going back to school, consider that many adults before you have overcome that feeling and opened up new worlds for themselves by doing so.

If you won't be returning to work or to school, you need to develop a meaningful structure in other ways. People often find that getting involved in volunteer activities can restore the sense of purpose to their lives, but only if they approach volunteering seriously and not as "busy work." When you volunteer, it's your precious time that is being committed, so choose involvements that allow you to develop new skills and to advance causes that are truly important to you.

The point is that to make pain management an integral part of your life, you have to keep growing. *When you sink into complacency, you sink, period.*

I never fail to marvel at what we can accomplish when we put aside disappointments and feel gratitude for the good things that have been given to us.

Open yourself up to gratitude and you will welcome every other strengthening quality as well. When you bring the people you love closer to you, you bring life itself closer to you. And there is no room for pain.

Reading List

Benson, H. 1975. *The Relaxation Response.* New York: William Morrow.

Bonica, J. J. 1990. *The Management of Pain.* Philadelphia: Lea & Febiger.

Burns, D. D. 1989. *The Feeling Good Handbook: Using the New Mood Therapy in Everyday Life.* New York: William Morrow.

Feldenkrais, M. 1972. *Awareness Through Movement: Health Exercises for Personal Growth.* New York: Harper & Row.

Kraus, H. 1988. *Diagnosis and Treatment of Muscle Pain.* Chicago: Quintessence Publishing Co.

Kraus, H. 1981. *The Sports Injury Book.* New York: Nick Lyons Books.

Lakein, A. 1974. *How to Get Control of Your Time and Your Life.* New York: New American Library.

Melzack, R., and Wall, P. D. 1988. *The Challenge of Pain.* New York: Penguin Books.

Peck, M. Scott. *The Road Less Traveled.* New York: Simon & Schuster, 1979.

Wall, P. D., and M. Jones. 1991. *Defeating Pain: The War Against a Silent Epidemic.* New York: Plenum Press.

Acknowledgments

Every successful pain management program depends on the skills and dedication of a wide variety of people. My own program is no different in this regard, but I am particularly fortunate, I think, in having a professional staff of such high caliber. Although only some of them are cited within the text, the influence of all of them is present. It is a pleasure to list here, with thanks for their contributions and cooperation, Karen Braglia, R.N.; Christina Casey, R.N.; Donald Douglas, M.D.; Michael Fox, P.T.; Barrie Guise, Ph.D.; Jorge Kirschtein, M.D.; Joan Leimbach, R.N.; Walter Matweychuk, Ph.D.; Dean Metz, P.T.; Pamela Picker, R.N.; Jane Prawda, O.T.; Lynn Savino, P.T.; Julie Weiner, and Eda Yuhjtman, P.T. I am also grateful for the tireless assistance of my dedicated support staff—Diana Ardrey, Cynthia Jones-Quartey, Maria Ortega, and Edna Perez—in providing information and documents.

My deepest appreciation goes to Allen Collins, M.D., for his encouragement and direction and to the administration of Lenox Hill Hospital for its vision in aiding in the establishment of my program.

A special thank-you to Hans Kraus, M.D., a pioneer in the treatment of chronic pain, who has played an important role in my life and my program and hence in the creation of this book.

Thanks also must go to my patients for giving me their trust and for showing me what courage can accomplish in the face of a seemingly intractable problem.

I have also been quite fortunate in my association with people who have helped me bring my message to the public. My thanks go to our editor, Fred Hills, for his endless enthusiasm, insightful comments, and skillful editing and to our agents, Herb and Nancy Katz, for defining the need for this book and for their invaluable assistance at every stage of its development. Jean Arbeiter's husband, Solomon, also merits gratitude for his patience and support.

Finally—but first in my heart—my thanks go to my wife, Suzy, not only for reading every word of the manuscript, but also for loving me along every step of the road we have traveled together.

Illustrations by Peg Gerrity
Diagrams by Janet Kroenke

Index